published by arrangement with **Gower Medical Publishing** · London · New York

SURGICAL ANATOMY OF THE HEART

Benson R. Wilcox, MD
Professor of Surgery
Chief, Division of Cardiothoracic Surgery
University of North Carolina
Chapel Hill, North Carolina, USA

Robert H. Anderson, BSc, MD, MRCPath
Joseph Levy Professor of Paediatric Cardiac Morphology
Cardiothoracic Institute
University of London
Honorary Consultant
The Brompton Hospital
London, UK

with forewords by

David C. Sabiston, Jr. MD
James Buchanan Duke Professor of Surgery and
Chairman of the Department
Duke University Medical Center
Durham, North Carolina

Thomas P. Graham, Jr. MD
Professor of Pediatrics and Director
Division of Pediatric Cardiology
Vanderbilt Medical Center
Nashville, Tennessee

Raven Press · New York

Distributed in the USA and Canada by:
Raven Press
1140 Avenue of the Americas
New York, New York 10036, USA

Distributed in all countries except USA, Canada and Japan by:
Churchill Livingstone
Robert Stevenson House
1-3 Baxter's Place
Leith Walk
Edinburgh EH1 3AF

Distributed in Japan by:
Nankodo Co., Ltd.
Tokyo International
P.O. Box 5272 (Mailing)
42-6, Hongo 3-chome
Bunkyo-ku
Tokyo 113, Japan

Library of Congress Catalog Card Number: 85-042754

Library Cataloging in Publication Data:
  Wilcox, B.
    Surgical anatomy of the heart.
    1. Heart – Anatomy
    I. Title II. Anderson, Robert H. (Robert Henry),
    1942
    611′.12 QM181

ISBN: 0-906923-22-0 (Gower)
          0-88167-103-7 (Raven Press)

Printed in Hong Kong by Mandarin Offset Marketing (H.K.) Ltd.

Project Editor: **Sharyn Wong**

Design: **Mehmet Hussein**
Robin Nicholl

Illustration: **Robin Nicholl**
Chris Furey

To our families:
Lucinda, Adelaide, Sandra, Melissa and Reid Wilcox;
Christine, Elizabeth and John Anderson

Preface

The books and articles devoted to technique in cardiac surgery are legion. This is most appropriate, since the success of cardiac surgery is greatly dependent upon excellent operative technique. But excellence of technique can be dissipated without a firm knowledge of the underlying cardiac morphology. This is as true for the 'normal heart' as for those hearts with complex congenital lesions. It is the feasibility of operating upon such complex malformations which has highlighted the need for a more detailed understanding of the basic anatomy in itself. Thus, in recent years surgeons have come to appreciate the necessity of avoiding damage to the coronary vessels, often invisible when working within the cardiac chambers, and particularly to the vital conduction tissues, invisible at all times. Although detailed and accurate descriptions of the conduction system have been available since the time of their discovery, only rarely have their positions been described with the cardiac surgeon in mind. Indeed, to the best of our knowledge there are no books which specifically display the anatomy of normal and abnormal hearts as perceived at the time of operation.

In writing this book we have tried to satisfy this need by combining the experience of a practising cardiac surgeon with that of a professional cardiac anatomist. We have emphasized the significant advances made in the last decade in appreciating the value of a detailed knowledge of cardiac anatomy. It is also our hope that the book will be of interest not only to the surgeon, but also the cardiologist, anaesthesiologist and surgical pathologist who ideally should have some knowledge of cardiac structures and its exquisite intricacies. Where appropriate, we have displayed our illustrations as seen by the surgeon, in many cases using material obtained in the operating room. To clarify the various orientations of each illustration, we have included a set of axes showing the directions of superior (S), inferior (I), anterior (A), posterior (P), left (L) and right (R). All our accounts are based on the anatomy as it is observed and, except in the case of aortic arch malformations, owe nothing to speculative embryology.

Acknowledgements

Both the material displayed in these pages and the concepts espoused are due in no small part to the help of our friends and collaborators. We owe a particular debt to Anton Becker of the University of Amsterdam who permitted us to use much of the material from his extensive collection of normal and pathological specimens. We have acknowledged our other friends at the appropriate point in the text, but here we would like to thank particularly Fergus Macartney of the Hospital for Sick Children, London, U.K.; Jim Wilkinson and Audrey Smith of the Institute of Child Health, Liverpool, U.K. and Bob Zuberbuhler of Pittsburgh Children's Hospital, Pennsylvania, U.S.A. The photographs and artwork could not have been produced without the considerable help given by Siew Yen Ho of the Cardiothoracic Institute and Charles Wright and his staff in the Department of Medical Illustration, University of North Carolina. We are indebted to Felicity Gil, Christine Anderson and Betsy Mann for their help during the preparation of the manuscript.

In all ventures of this kind, a debt is due to colleagues who shoulder the burden when our minds are on writing rather than on other responsibilities. In this respect we thank Gordon Murray, Peter Starek and Blair Keagy of the University of North Carolina. The experience gained in studying the malformed hearts would have been impossible without the support of other colleagues, and here we thank Christopher Lincoln, Elliot Shinebourne, Michael Joseph and Graham Miller of the Brompton Hospital. Finally, it is a pleasure to acknowledge the support of Gower Medical Publishing, who turned an often untidy manuscript into, in our opinion, a beautiful work of art.

B.R.W. & R.H.A.
Chapel Hill, 1985

Foreword A Clinician's View

It is a great pleasure for me to write a foreword to this beautiful demonstration of anatomy of the normal and the congenitally malformed heart. Drs. Wilcox and Anderson, along with their collaborating colleagues, have produced a book which I would classify as 'must reading' for the clinician who cares for the very young as well as the older child or adult patient with congenital heart disease. As clinicians we are used to images that are somewhat remote from the source, even though the current imaging modalities can give us exquisite detail on most occasions. Radiographic, echocardiographic and angiographic anatomy provide the 'road maps' that we use in attempting to classify and then manage patients with congenital cardiac anomalies. The accuracy with which these images represent the anatomical detail seen in the operating room provides the true test of the usefulness of any of these procedures. All too often the clinician does not venture into the operating room in order to appreciate the fact that the exposed beating heart is not as clearly delineated in all its details as one would picture from the usual textbook illustrations and as one would imagine from viewing angiographic and echocardiographic anatomy.

The illustrations presented in this book are truly outstanding in demonstrating the surgical anatomy of the heart and in relating this to easy-to-read diagrammatic representations of the important anatomical landmarks as well as to practical and useful nomenclature. The text is written clearly and lucidly with sufficient detail but it does not approach the redundant or the tedious.

I can recommend this book highly and without reservation for all trainees and practitioners of the art of clinical cardiology as it applies to patients with congenital heart defects. My congratulations to Drs. Wilcox and Anderson.

T.P. Graham, Jr.
Nashville

Foreword

Since the advent of cardiac surgery, and more especially of surgical procedures on the open heart, the importance of a fundamental understanding of anatomical details concerning congenital malformations and pathological changes has been of great significance. Of special importance are the variations which occur and the inclusion of adequate illustrative material to make the points with emphasis and conviction. Drs. Wilcox and Anderson have brilliantly achieved these features in their remarkable **Surgical Anatomy of the Heart**. They have had the foresight to study carefully their own anatomical collections and, in addition, have sought specimens from other outstanding collections both in the United Kingdom and in the United States. These combine to make a hitherto unavailable reference source which can only be described in the most superlative terms.

The authors initiate this beautiful collection with a chapter on surgical approaches to the heart, with emphasis upon significant features of the chest wall and of the vessels and nerves which course through the mediastinum and thoracic cavity. Special emphasis is given to median sternotomy, since it is the most common of the currently employed incisions to expose the heart. The comments about the internal mammary artery and the phrenic nerve are particularly appropriate.

The next chapter reviews in appropriate detail the surgical anatomy of the normal heart, a section which is of singular importance. A firm knowledge of the normal heart is obviously necessary in order to understand the abnormal anatomy. These features are beautifully achieved by the color plates. The authors have omitted labelling the color photographs, which might mar their meaningfulness, by electing rather to place beside the color plates a diagram with the appropriate labelling. Examples of the impact of this section include superb illustrations of the triangle of Koch with its physiological implications in cardiac conduction. Similarly, valvar attachments are brilliantly depicted. While the majority of the diagrammatic illustrations are in black and white, colors are also used effectively to supplement the illustrative impressions.

The next chapter considers the surgical anatomy of the coronary circulation, a subject of ever increasing importance in both acquired and congenital heart disease. The variations which occur in the coronary arteries are assuming increasing significance, and a knowledge of these patterns is essential for appropriate interpretation of both coronary arteriograms and of the operative anatomy at the time of myocardial revascularization. The intimate relationship of a dominant left coronary artery to the mitral valve ring, for example, is convincingly depicted and described. This section is quite comprehensive with detailed consideration of the position of the retrocaval sinus node artery relative to the oval fossa and to the terminal crest. Consideration is also devoted to anomalous origin of the left coronary artery from the pulmonary artery, a malformation which is being recognized with increasing frequency.

In keeping with diagnostic and surgical strides in the field of cardiac dysrhythmias, a very thoughtful chapter is devoted to the surgical anatomy of the conduction system. The illustrations which comprise this section are the best this reviewer has seen and are presented in a very lucid manner. Detailed consideration of the accessory atrioventricular pathways which produce the Wolff-Parkinson-White syndrome are precisely described and illustrated with emphasis upon the fact that these pathways are often inappropriately termed 'bundles of Kent'. These pathways can be found anywhere around the atrioventricular junction and can be categorized as left-sided, right-sided, and septal pathways. Emphasis is placed upon the fact that the anatomical features of each group show significant differences.

The section which follows is unique in that it comprises an analytic description of congenitally malformed hearts with primary attention directed toward the anatomic lesions without undue reference to embryological concepts, especially when the latter are primarily theoretical. In other words, it is recognized that the prime feature of a cardiac malformation rests not with its presumed embryological development, but rather in the precise facts surrounding its basic anatomy. Thus, the authors present a clinically useful system with accurate descriptions in the finest detail. In this section, ambiguous atrioventricular connections should be cited as a prime example and again are superbly illustrated, leaving the reader with a deep sense of conviction of their accuracy. The conduction system is again emphasized for each of the malformations with considerations of the variations which occur.

The beauty of the organization of this unique monograph is further illustrated by the chapter which concerns lesions in normally connected hearts. The various congenital malformations are then considered, beginning with the simplest and progressing to the most complex. It is here that the details of the diagrams, side-by-side with the color photographs, become most impressive. Moreover, a number of these were obtained intraoperatively and thereby emphasize in a special way their meaningfulness to cardiac surgeons. When preserved specimens are used they are also well illustrated and capture the primary points exceedingly well. It is a comprehensive work and one which is directed towards making certain that the reader fully

comprehends the message being transmitted. This chapter is followed by one considering, in the same manner, lesions in abnormally connected hearts, including the double inlet ventricle, absent atrioventricular connection (tricuspid atresia), complete transposition and congenitally corrected transposition. Double outlet right ventricle and common arterial trunk are also precisely illustrated, together with their variations.

Abnormalities of the great vessels are considered in a separate chapter which is characterized by completeness. In sequential order, malformations of the systemic and pulmonary veins, the thoracic aorta, the patency of the arterial duct, and aorto-pulmonary window are presented. The authors have made astute choices of illustrations and, as in all sections of this book, the emphasis is placed upon the fundamental principles to grasp as well as the anatomic details.

The final chapter concerns positional anomalies of the heart with the recognition that surgical problems posed by cardiac malformation are often accentuated when the heart is in an abnormal position. This concept presents an approach which is seldom emphasized, but is of considerable significance as simple review of the pertinent points becomes rapidly convincing for the reader. This is most vividly underscored in considering deformities such as ectopia cordis and the anatomic configurations which are paramount in successful surgical correction.

In summary, **Surgical Anatomy of the Heart** provides the reader with an entirely new experience in combining anatomical and physiological concepts through expertly selected color plates of the specimens, each with accompanying labelled diagrams and narrative. Gower Medical Publishing is deserving of special praise for their extraordinary reproduction of the illustrations and attractive arrangement of the entire text. Such an array of unique illustrations and carefully chosen narrative has not been previously available. For these reasons, this monograph will predictably become an essential feature in the libraries of cardiac surgeons and cardiologists alike. Moreover, it has an even wider impact including its relevance to radiologists and pathologists, and to all those who encounter problems relating to disorders of the heart. It is a masterful work and one which will surely be cited in scholarly works of the future. The authors deserve great admiration and praise for the painstaking way in which they have produced this book, and equally they can be assured that this work will be enthusiastically received and will long endure as a landmark in the field.

David C. Sabiston, Jr.
Durham   vii

Contents

1 Surgical Approaches to the Heart

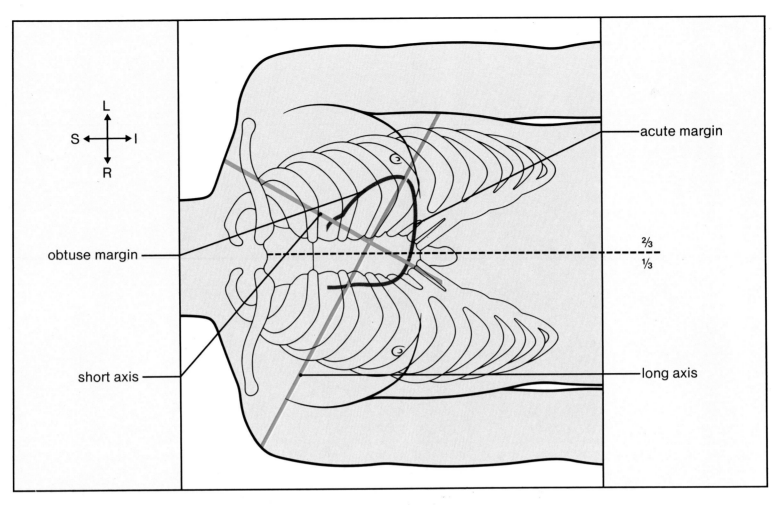

Fig. 1.1 *Usual position of the heart within the thorax showing vital landmarks and areas as seen with the patient supine on the operating table.*

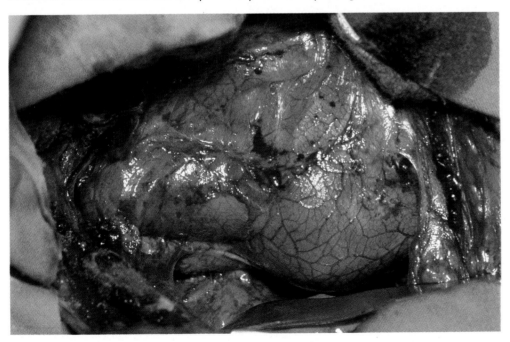

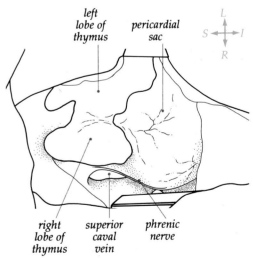

Fig. 1.2 *Operative view of the extent of the thymus gland in an infant.*

The heart lies in the mediastinum in the normal individual with two-thirds of its bulk to the left of the midline (Fig. 1.1). The heart and great vessels can therefore be approached either through the thoracic cavity or directly through the midline anteriorly. To make such approaches safely, knowledge is required of the salient anatomical features of the chest wall and of the other vessels and nerves which course through the mediastinum.

The most frequently used approach is a median sternotomy. The soft tissue incision is made in the midline and extends from the suprasternal notch to below the xiphoid process. Inferiorly the linea alba is incised between the two rectus sheaths, taking care to avoid entry to the peritoneal cavity or damage to an enlarged liver if present. Reflection of the origin of the rectus muscles in this area reveals the xiphoid process which can be

incised to provide access to the anterior mediastinum. Superiorly a vertical incision is made between the sternal insertions of the sternocleidomastoid muscles; this exposes the relatively bloodless midline raphe between the right and left sternohyoid and sternothyroid muscles. An incision through this raphe then gives access to the superior aspect of the anterior mediastinum. The anterior mediastinum immediately behind the

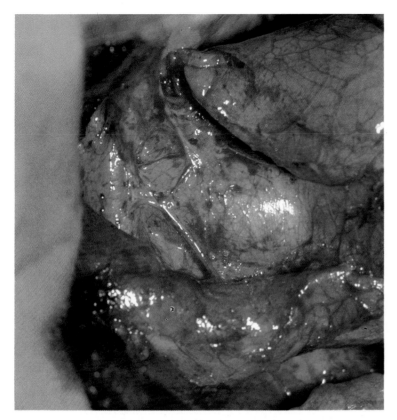

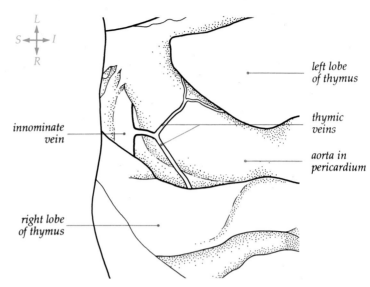

Fig. 1.3 *Operative view of the delicate veins which drain from the thymus to the left brachiocephalic vein.*

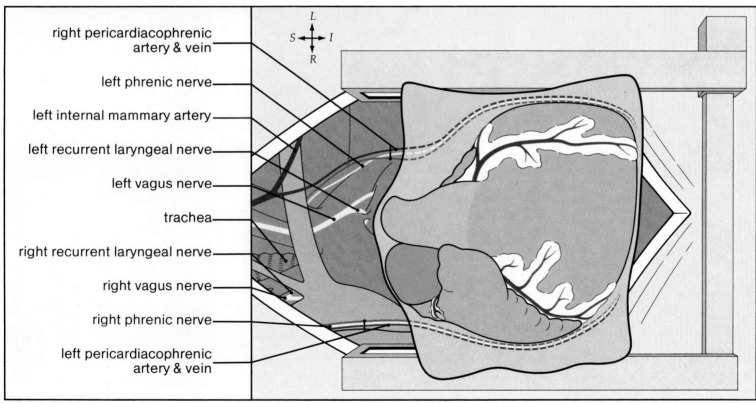

right pericardiacophrenic
artery & vein

left phrenic nerve

left internal mammary artery

left recurrent laryngeal nerve

left vagus nerve

trachea

right recurrent laryngeal nerve

right vagus nerve

right phrenic nerve

left pericardiacophrenic
artery & vein

Fig. 1.4 *Surgical view through a median sternotomy with the pericardium opened showing the phrenic and vagus nerves to be well clear of the operative field.*

sternum is devoid of vital structures so that these two incisions can safely be joined by blunt dissection in the retrosternal space. When the sternum has been split, retraction will reveal the pericardial sac lying between the pleural cavities. Superiorly the thymus gland wraps itself over the anterior and lateral aspects of the pericardium in the area of exit of the great arteries, the gland being a particularly prominent structure in the

infant (Fig. 1.2). It has two lateral lobes joined more or less in the midline which sometimes must be divided or partially excised to provide adequate exposure. The arterial supply to the thymus is from the internal thoracic (mammary) and inferior thyroid arteries. If divided, these arteries tend to retreat beneath the sternum and can produce troublesome bleeding. The veins are fragile, often emptying into the left innominate

(brachiocephalic) vein via a common trunk (Fig. 1.3). Undue traction on the gland can lead to damage to this major vessel.

Having exposed the pericardial sac within the mediastinum, gaining access to the heart should not pose any problem. The vagus and phrenic nerves traverse the length of the pericardium but are well lateral (Fig. 1.4). The phrenic nerve on each side passes anterior and the vagus nerve posterior to the hilum of the lung.

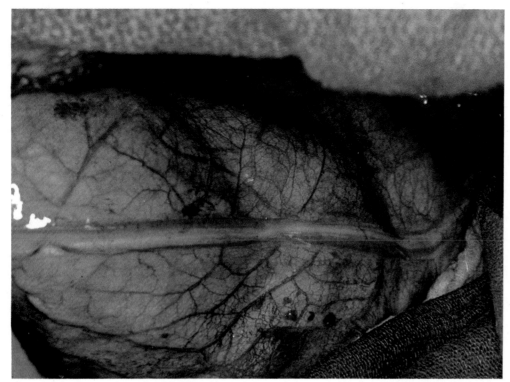

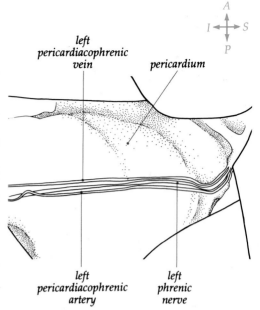

left
pericardiacophrenic
vein

pericardium

left
pericardiacophrenic
artery

left
phrenic
nerve

Fig. 1.5 *Operative view through a left lateral thoracotomy of the left phrenic nerve coursing over the pericardium.*

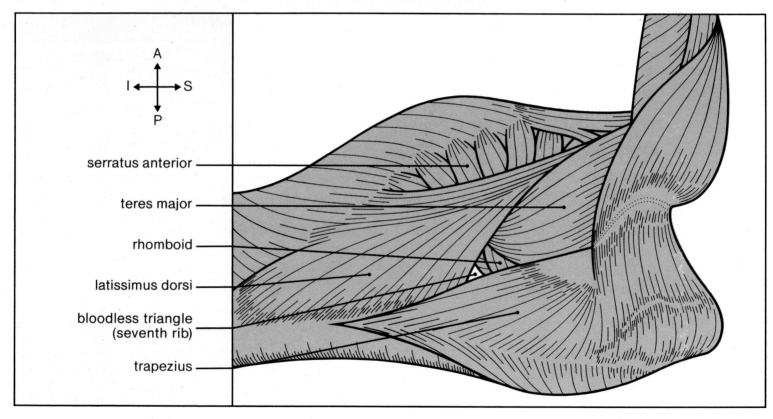

serratus anterior

teres major

rhomboid

latissimus dorsi

bloodless triangle
(seventh rib)

trapezius

Fig. 1.6 *The bloodless area overlying the posterior extent of the sixth intercostal space.*

These nerves are much more at risk during lateral thoracotomies (Fig. 1.5) but can be damaged by injudicious use of cooling agents within the pericardial cavity. The phrenic nerves are also vulnerable when pericardium is harvested for use as an intracardiac patch or baffle. As they traverse the pericardium the phrenic nerves are accompanied by the pericardiacophrenic arteries, branches of the internal thoracic arteries. These should not be at risk with a median sternotomy, but the pericardiacophrenic

origin can be avulsed by excessive traction. The internal thoracic arteries themselves are more liable to injury during closure of the incision.

Standard lateral thoracotomies provide access to the heart and great vessels via the pleural spaces. Left-sided incisions provide ready access to the great arteries, pulmonary veins and left-sided heart chambers. Most frequently the incision is made in the fourth intercostal space. The posterior extent is through the triangular, relatively bloodless, space between the

edges of the latissimus dorsi, trapezius and teres major muscles (Fig. 1.6). The floor of this triangle is the sixth intercostal space. Division of latissimus dorsi and a portion of trapezius posteriorly, together with serratus anteriorly, frees the scapula so that the fourth intercostal space can be identified. Its precise identity should be confirmed by counting down from above. The intercostal muscles are then divided equidistant between the fourth and fifth ribs. The incision is carried forward to about the midclavicular line in

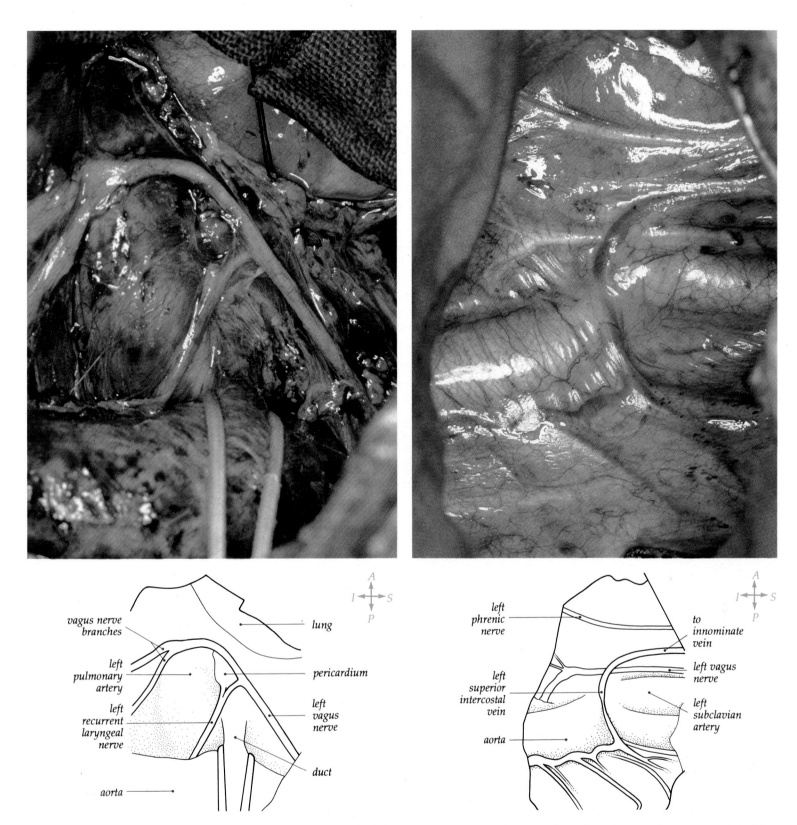

Fig. 1.7 *Operative view through a left lateral thoracotomy of the left recurrent laryngeal nerve passing round the duct in an adult.*

Fig. 1.8 *Operative view through a left lateral thoracotomy of the left superior intercostal vein.*

submammary position, being careful to avoid damage to the nipple and breast tissue. The intercostal neurovascular bundle is well protected beneath the lower margin of the fourth rib. Having divided the musculature as far as the pleura, the pleural space is entered and the lung permitted to collapse away from the chest wall. Posterior retraction of the lung reveals the middle mediastinum with the left lateral lobe of the thymus overlying the pericardial sac and aortic arch with its associated nerves and

vessels. Intrapericardial access is usually gained anterior to the phrenic nerve. On occasion the thymus may require elevation when the incision is extended superiorly and then the same precautions should be taken as discussed above.
To approach the aortic isthmus and descending thoracic aorta, the lung is retracted anteriorly and the parietal pleura divided on its mediastinal aspect. Usually this is done posterior to the vagus nerve. In this area the vagus gives off the left recurrent laryngeal nerve which passes

round the inferior border of the arterial ligament (or duct) (Fig. 1.7) to ascend towards the larynx on the medial aspect of the posterior wall of the aorta. Excessive traction of the vagus nerve as it courses into the thorax along the left subclavian artery can cause injury to the recurrent laryngeal nerve just as readily as direct trauma to the nerve in the environs of the ligament. The superior intercostal vein is seen crossing the aorta and insinuating itself between the phrenic and vagus nerves (Fig. 1.8), but this structure is

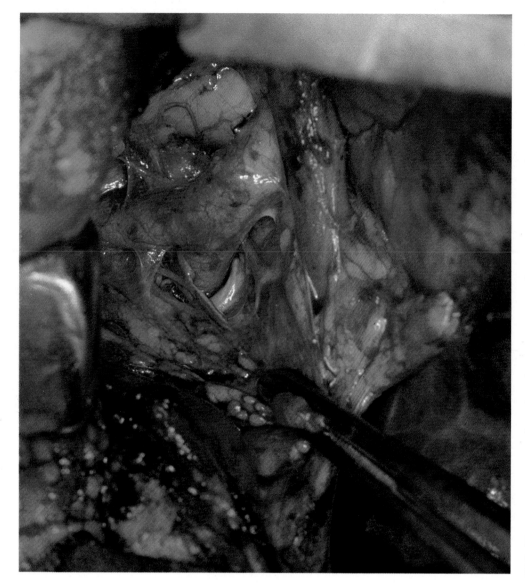

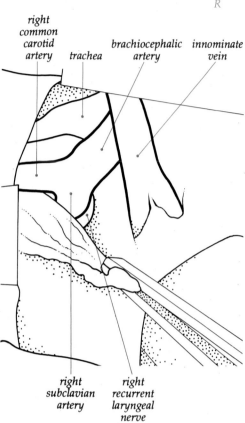

right
common
carotid
artery   trachea   brachiocephalic   innominate
                      artery   vein

right   right
subclavian   recurrent
artery   laryngeal
                      nerve

Fig. 1.9 *Operative view through a median sternotomy of the origin of the right recurrent laryngeal nerve.*

rarely of surgical significance. The thoracic duct ascends medially through this area to drain into the left subclavian vein at its junction with the internal jugular. Accessory lymph channels draining into the duct can be troublesome when dissecting the origin of the left subclavian artery.

A right thoracotomy is made through an incision similar to that for a left thoracotomy in either the fourth or fifth interspace. The fifth interspace is used when approaching the heart and the fourth to gain access to the right-sided great vessels. Access to the pericardium is gained by incising anterior to the phrenic

nerve, often necessitating retraction of the right lobe of the thymus. To reach the right pulmonary artery and adjacent mediastinal structures, it is sometimes useful to divide the azygos vein near its junction with the superior caval vein. Extension of this incision superiorly exposes the origin of the right subclavian branch of the brachiocephalic (innominate) trunk. Laterally this artery is crossed by the right vagus nerve, the right recurrent laryngeal nerve taking off from the vagus and curling round the posteroinferior wall of the artery before ascending into the neck (Fig. 1.9). Also encircling the subclavian origin on this

right side is the subclavian sympathetic loop (ansa subclavia), a branch of the sympathetic trunk which runs up into the neck. Damage to this structure can result in Horner's syndrome.

In treating congenital heart disease, anterior right or left thoracotomies would only rarely be used. Once the chest is opened, the same basic anatomical rules apply as described above.

Thus far, our account has presumed the presence of normal anatomy. In many instances, the cardiac disposition is altered by the congenital anomaly present. These alterations will be described in the appropriate sections.

2 Surgical Anatomy of the Normal Heart

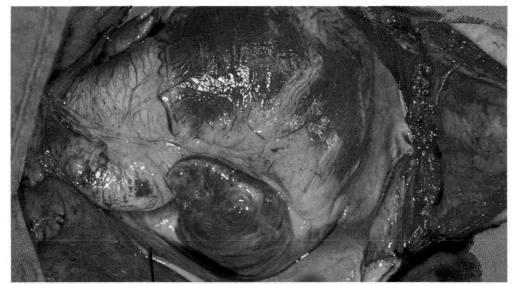

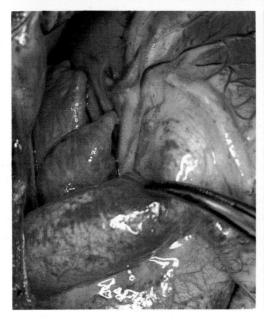

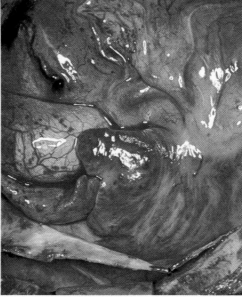

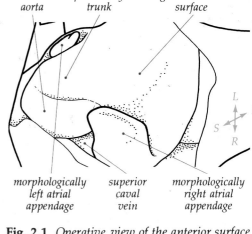

Fig. 2.1 *Operative view of the anterior surface of the heart following incision of the pericardium.*

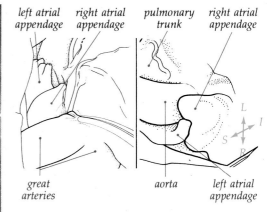

Fig. 2.2 *Juxtaposition of atrial appendages: (left) complete transposition and left juxtaposition; (right) origin of the left coronary artery from the pulmonary trunk and right juxtaposition, both seen through a median sternotomy.*

When we describe the heart in this and subsequent chapters, the terms used will be relative to the heart in the anatomical position. However, whenever possible we will illustrate the heart as it would be viewed by the surgeon during an operative procedure. Where we illustrate the heart in more 'pathological' views, this will be clearly stated.

Regardless of the surgical approach, having entered the mediastinum the surgeon will be confronted by the heart enclosed in its pericardial sac. Although in the strict sense the pericardial sac has two layers, from a practical point of view it is made up of the tough fibrous pericardium. This fibrous sac encloses the mass of the heart and, by virtue of its own attachments to the diaphragm, helps support the position of the heart within the mediastinum. The sac is free-standing around the atrial and ventricular chambers but becomes adherent to the adventitia of the great arteries and veins at their entrances to and exits from the heart, these attachments closing the pericardial cavity. The pericardial cavity itself is contained between the two layers of serous pericardium, a thin-walled double-

layered sac which exists within the fibrous cavity. Because the outer layer of the serous pericardium is densely adherent to the fibrous pericardium, and because the inner layer is the epicardium, the pericardial cavity is in essence the space between the fibrous pericardium and the surface of the heart. By virtue of the shape of the cardiac chambers and great arteries, there are two recesses within the pericardial cavity which are lined by serous pericardium. The first is the transverse sinus which occupies the inner curvature of the heart. Anteriorly it is bounded by the posterior surface of the great arteries; posteriorly it is limited by the anterior interatrial groove. The sinus is a curved tube-like space with a recess between the superior caval vein and the right upper pulmonary vein. The right lateral border of this recess is a pericardial fold between the superior caval vein and the right upper pulmonary vein. Incisions through this fold provide good access to the superior aspect of the left atrium and the right pulmonary artery as it curves posteriorly towards the hilum of the lung. Laterally on each side, the ends of the transverse sinus are in free

communication with the rest of the pericardial cavity.

The second pericardial recess is the oblique sinus, a cul-de-sac behind the left atrium. The upper boundary of this space is formed by the reflection of serous pericardium between the upper pulmonary veins at their entrance to the left atrium. The right border is the reflection of pericardium around the right pulmonary veins and inferior caval vein. To the left is found the reflection of pericardium around the left pulmonary veins. With the usual surgical approach through a median sternotomy the fibrous pericardium is opened more or less in the midline and retracted laterally, exposing the anterior surface of the heart and great vessels (Fig. 2.1). It is worthwhile noting the external features of the heart as revealed by this approach. The pulmonary trunk and aorta leave the base of the heart and extend in a superior direction, with the aortic root in posterior and rightward position. An anomalous position of the aortic root almost always indicates abnormal ventriculoarterial connexions (see Chapter 7). The atrial appendages may be seen one to either side of the

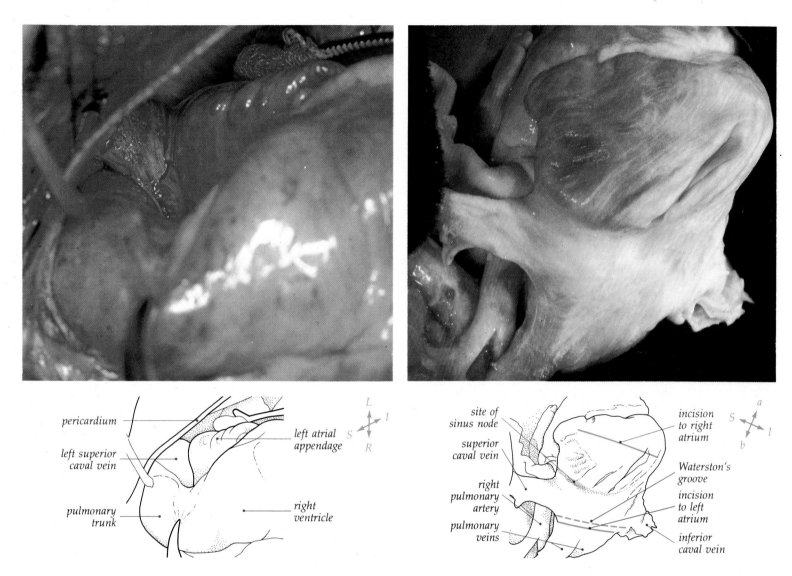

Fig. 2.3 *A left superior caval vein seen through a median sternotomy as it dips between the left appendage and left pulmonary artery. The pulmonary trunk is retracted to the right.*

Fig. 2.4 *Terminal sulcus and site of Waterston's groove in surgical orientation. Note superimposition of possible incisions to the right and left atria and position of the sinus node.*

prominent arterial pedicle. The morphologically right appendage is more prominent and has a blunt triangular shape. The morphologically left appendage may not be seen immediately. If searched for at the left border of the pulmonary trunk it will be found to be a narrow crennellated structure. Presence of the two appendages on the same side of the arterial pedicle is an anomaly in itself (juxtaposition of the atrial appendages). Left juxtaposition (both appendages to the left of the arterial pedicle) is always found in the presence of other severe malformations, particularly abnormal ventriculoarterial connexions (Fig. 2.2, left) (*Melhuish & Van Praagh, 1968*; see Chapter 7). However, the much rarer right juxtaposition (Fig. 2.2, right) can be found with normal chamber connexions, but it too can exist with complex congenital heart disease (*Anderson, Smith & Wilkinson, 1976*). While inspecting the left border of the heart it is also of value to search for a persistent left superior caval vein. When present, this venous channel indents the pericardial cavity between the anterior left atrial appendage and the posterior left pulmonary veins. Within the cavity it lies between the left appendage and the left

pulmonary artery (Fig. 2.3).

The ventricular mass extends from the base of the heart to the apex and its axis usually extends into the left hemithorax. An anomalous position of either the ventricular mass or the apex is again highly suggestive of the presence of congenital cardiac malformation (see Chapter 9). In shape the ventricular mass is a three-sided pyramid, having diaphragmatic, anterior (sternocostal) and left (pulmonary) surfaces. The margin between the first two surfaces is sharp, the acute (right) margin. The transition between the latter two surfaces is more gradual, the obtuse margin. The greater part of the anterior surface of the ventricular mass is occupied by the morphologically right ventricle. Its left border, close to the obtuse margin, is marked by the anterior interventricular (descending) branch of the left coronary artery, which curves onto the ventricular surface between the left atrial appendage and the basal origin of the pulmonary trunk. The right border of the morphologically right ventricle is marked by the right coronary artery running obliquely in the atrioventricular sulcus. Unusually prominent coronary arteries coursing

onto the ventricular surface between these two arteries should raise the suspicion of significant cardiac malformations.

The surface anatomy of the heart is significant in determining the most appropriate site for an incision to gain access to a given cardiac chamber. For example, the relatively bloodless outlet portion of the right ventricle just beneath the origin of the pulmonary trunk affords ready access to the right ventricular cavity. The important landmark for the right atrium is the terminal sulcus between the appendage and the venous component (Fig. 2.4), the vital structure in this area being the sinus node located at the lateral superior cavoatrial junction. The important artery to the sinus node can also be seen on occasion as it either crosses the crest of the right appendage or courses retrocavally to enter the terminal sulcus between the superior and inferior caval orifices. Posterior and parallel to the terminal sulcus is a second deeper groove between the right atrium and the right pulmonary veins (Waterston's groove). This groove serves as a guide for surgical incisions into the left atrium (Fig. 2.4).

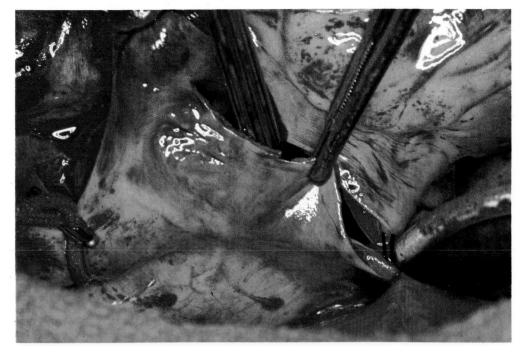

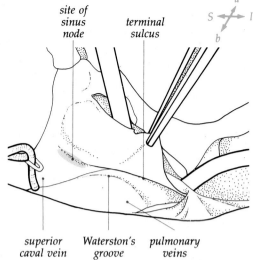

site of
sinus
node

terminal
sulcus

superior
caval vein

Waterston's
groove

pulmonary
veins

Fig. 2.5 *Operative view of the terminal sulcus, site of the sinus node and a safe incision into the right atrium.*

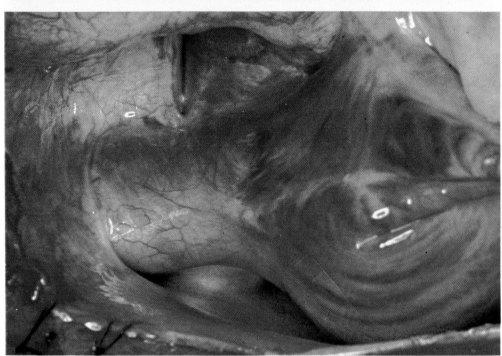

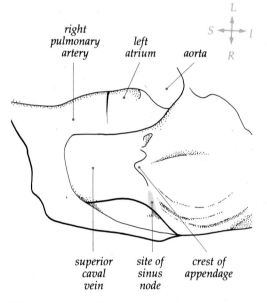

right
pulmonary
artery

left
atrium

aorta

superior
caval
vein

site of
sinus
node

crest of
appendage

Fig. 2.6 *Operative view of the crest of the right atrial appendage with the position of the sinus node superimposed.*

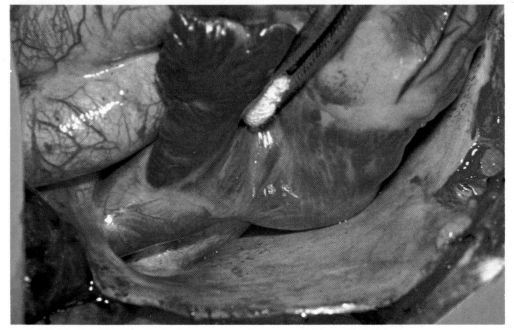

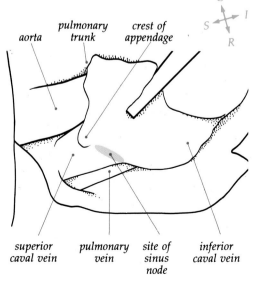

aorta

pulmonary
trunk

crest of
appendage

superior
caval vein

pulmonary
vein

site of
sinus
node

inferior
caval vein

Fig. 2.7 *Operative view of the terminal sulcus and site of the sinus node.*

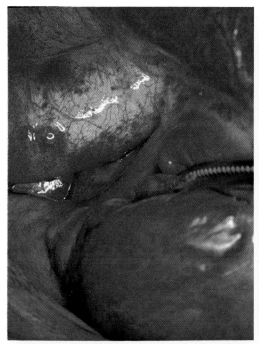
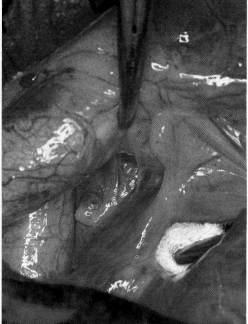
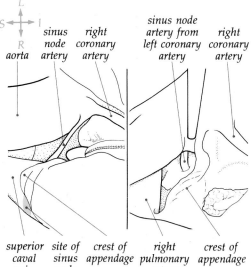

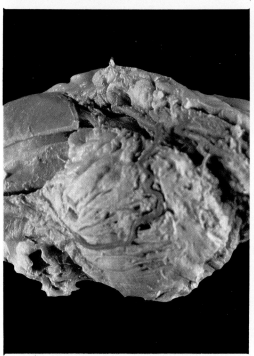
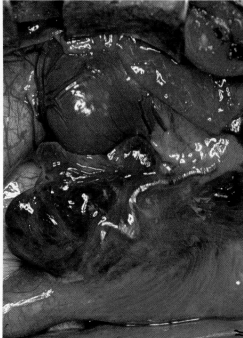
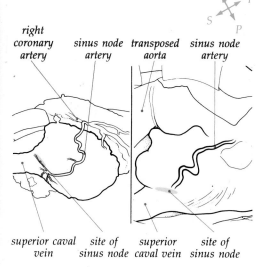

Fig. 2.8 *Operative views of origin of the sinus node artery (left) from the right coronary artery and (right) from the left coronary artery.*

Fig. 2.9 *Anomalous course of the sinus node artery as demonstrated by dissection (left) and as seen at surgery (right). Left by courtesy of Prof. F. Fontan & Mr. J. Busquet.*

i. Morphologically right atrium

The right atrium has two basic parts, the appendage and the venous sinus, the latter receiving the systemic venous return. As we have indicated, the junction of the two parts is identified by the presence of a prominent groove, the terminal sulcus (Fig. 2.5). As also described, the appendage is an extensive structure of blunt triangular shape and has a wide junction with the venous sinus across the terminal sulcus. The venous sinus is much smaller when viewed externally, extending between the terminal sulcus and Waterston's groove. It receives the superior and inferior caval veins at its extremities (Fig. 2.4). Superiorly and anteriorly the appendage has a further important relation with the superior caval vein. Here the appendage terminates in a prominent crest which forms the summit of the

terminal sulcus and is continuous behind the aorta in the transverse sinus with the interatrial groove (Fig. 2.6). Almost always, the sinus node lies within the terminal sulcus in a subepicardial position. It is a spindle-shaped structure lying to the right of the crest, that is, lateral to the superior cavoatrial junction (Fig. 2.7). However, in about one-tenth of cases the node may extend across the crest into the interatrial groove, draping itself across the cavoatrial junction in horseshoe fashion (*Anderson, Ho & Anderson, 1979*).

Of equal surgical significance is the course of the important artery to the sinus node. This is said to be an initial branch of the right coronary artery in about 55 percent of individuals and a branch of the circumflex artery in the remainder (*James, 1961*). Irrespective of its origin, it usually

courses through the anterior interatrial groove towards the superior cavoatrial junction, frequently running within the atrial myocardium (Fig. 2.8). A significant variant is found when the artery originates from the right coronary artery some distance from the aorta and courses over the lateral surface of the appendage to reach the terminal sulcus (Fig. 2.9). This, however, is rare. Almost always the artery approaches the cavoatrial junction through the interatrial groove, but may then cross the crest of the appendage, course retrocavally or even divide to form an arterial circle round the junction. All these variations should be taken into account when planning the safest right atrial incision, particularly when the nodal artery crosses the lateral margin of the appendage.

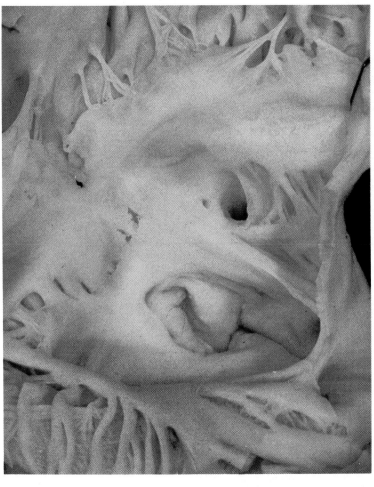

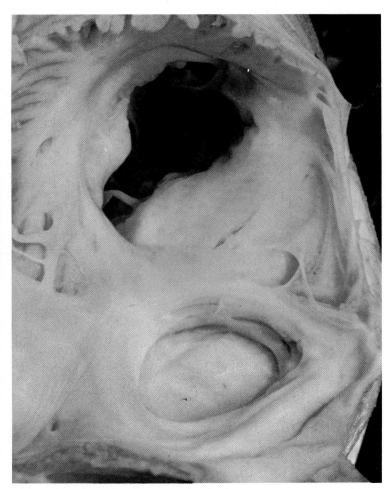

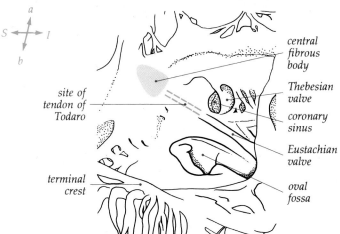

Fig. 2.10 *Landmarks of the atrial septum in surgical orientation.*

Fig. 2.11 *The apparently great expanse of the atrial septum in surgical orientation after removal of the superior caval vein.*

Opening the atrium through the best incision shows that the sulcus is the external marking of a prominent muscle bundle, the terminal crest, which separates the pectinate muscles of the appendage from the smooth walls of the venous sinus (Fig. 2.10). Anteriorly the crest curves in front of the orifice of the superior caval vein to become continuous with the so-called 'secondary septum' or the superior limbus of the oval fossa. On first sight when inspecting the right atrium through this incision there appears to be an extensive septal surface between the orifices of the caval veins and the orifice of the tricuspid valve (Fig. 2.11), but the apparent extent of this septum is spurious (*Sweeney & Rosenquist, 1979;*

Anderson & Becker, 1980a). Opening into and from this 'septal' surface are the oval fossa and the orifice of the coronary sinus. The true septum between the right and left atrial chambers is confined to the immediate environs of the oval fossa, as shown by the dissection in Fig. 2.12. The extensive 'secondary septum' or, as it is better termed, the superior limbus, is produced by folding of the interatrial groove between the venous sinus and the pulmonary veins. The inferior margin of the oval fossa is produced by another important muscle bundle, the sinus septum or inferior limbus. This bundle swings in from the terminal crest and separates the orifice of the inferior caval vein from that of the coronary sinus and

also separates the coronary sinus from the oval fossa (Fig. 2.13). Only that part of the inferior limbus immediately adjacent to the oval fossa is a true septal structure. Similarly only a small part of the extensive superior limbus separates the right from the left atrium. Its larger part is the atrial wall overlying the aortic root. These limited margins of the true atrial septum are of major surgical importance since it is an easy matter to pass outside the heart when attempting to gain access to the left atrium through a right atrial incision. In addition to the position of the sinus node and the extent of the atrial septum, the other major area of surgical significance in the morphologically right atrium is the site of the atrioventricular node.

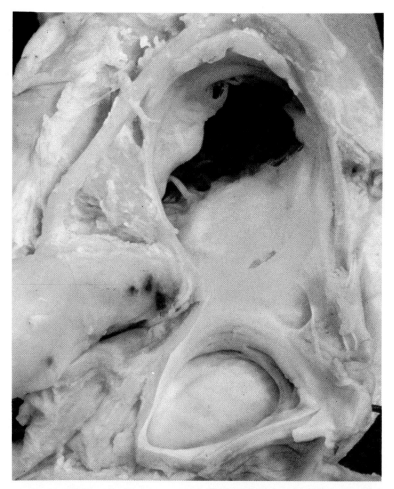

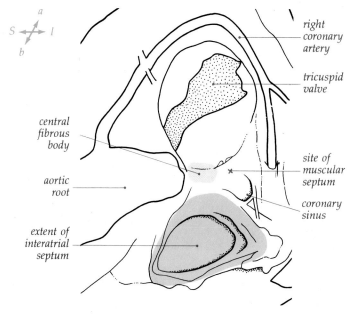

Fig. 2.12 *Further removal of all non-septal parts of the atrial wall above the oval fossa. Note how little of the 'septum' is a true interatrial structure.*

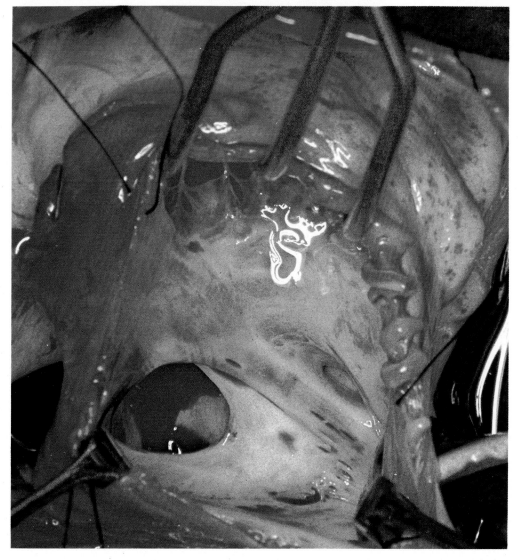

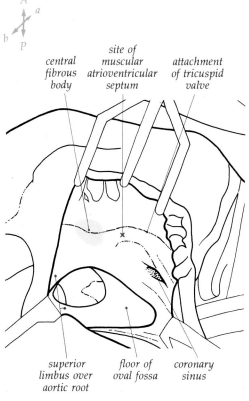

Fig. 2.13 *Operative view of the opened right atrium, with an atrial septal defect within the oval fossa, showing septal landmarks.*

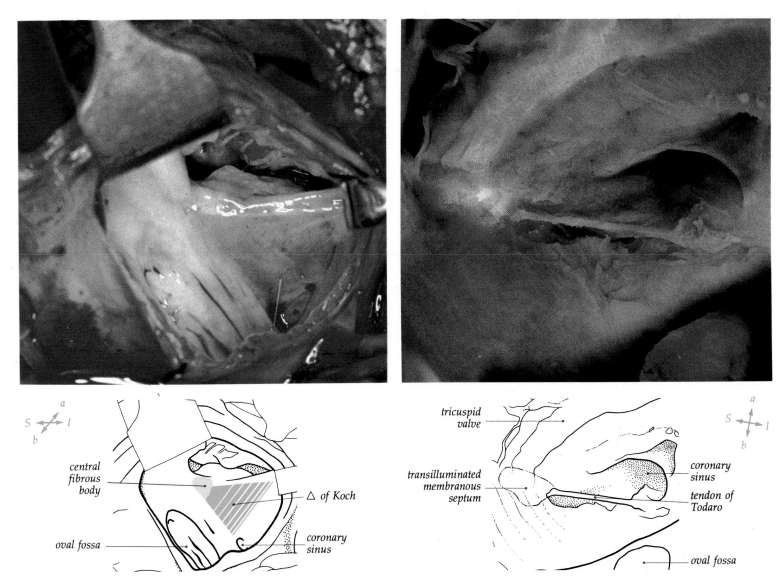

Fig. 2.14 *Operative view of the triangle of Koch.*

Fig. 2.15 *Tendon of Todaro with transillumination of the membranous septum and oval fossa. By courtesy of Prof. A.E. Becker, University of Amsterdam.*

This is contained within the triangle of Koch (Fig. 2.14). This important landmark is bounded by the tendon of Todaro, the attachment of the septal leaflet of the tricuspid valve and the orifice of the coronary sinus. The tendon of Todaro is a fibrous structure formed by the junction of the Eustachian valve (valve of the inferior caval vein) and the Thebesian valve (valve of the coronary sinus). The commissure of these two valvar structures buries itself in the sinus septum and runs forward as the tendon of Todaro to insert into the central fibrous body (Fig. 2.15). The entire atrial component of the atrioventricular conduction tissues is contained within the confines of the triangle of Koch. If this area is scrupulously avoided during surgical procedures, the atrioventricular conduction tissues cannot be damaged. Should the node need to be precisely identified, it should be remembered that the tricuspid valve attachment is some way down the surface of the septum relative to the mitral valve attachment (Fig. 2.16). The node itself, sitting in interatrial position on the sloping face of the atrioventricular muscular septum, is therefore some distance above the tricuspid valve attachment. The atrioventricular bundle, however, penetrates more or less directly at the apex of the triangle of Koch.

Much has been written in recent years concerning the role of 'specialized' pathways of tissue in conduction of the sinus impulse to the atrioventricular node. Indeed, some surgical operations have been specially modified to avoid these presumed tracts. From the anatomical standpoint it can now be stated unequivocally that there are no insulated, isolated tracts between the nodes to be avoided at surgery as one might avoid the penetrating and branching atrioventricular bundle (*Anderson et al., 1981*). In the atria the major muscle bundles serve as preferential pathways of conduction, but the course of these preferential pathways is dictated by overall atrial geometry. Ideally, prominent muscle bundles such as the terminal crest, the superior limbus or the sinus septum should be preserved during atrial surgery; but even if they cannot be preserved, the surgeon can rest assured that internodal conduction will continue as long as some strand of atrial myocardium connects the nodes and providing that nodal arteries or the nodes themselves are not traumatized. The key to avoiding atrial arrhythmias is the fastidious preservation of the sinus and atrioventricular nodes and their arteries, rather than worrying about non-existent tracts of 'specialized atrial conduction tissues'.

The tricuspid orifice, the vestibule to the right ventricle, is continuous with both parts of the right atrium, the venous sinus and the appendage. The anterior junction of these two parts overlies the anteroseptal commissure of the valve and the supra-ventricular crest of the right ventricle. The posterior junction is at the orifice of the coronary sinus, where there is usually an extensive trabeculated diverticulum found behind the sinus, the so-called post-Eustachian sinus of Keith (Fig. 2.17).

Although it is not always easy, it is generally possible to distinguish three leaflets in the tricuspid valve orifice: the anterosuperior, the septal, and the inferior or mural leaflet (Figs. 2.17 & 2.18).

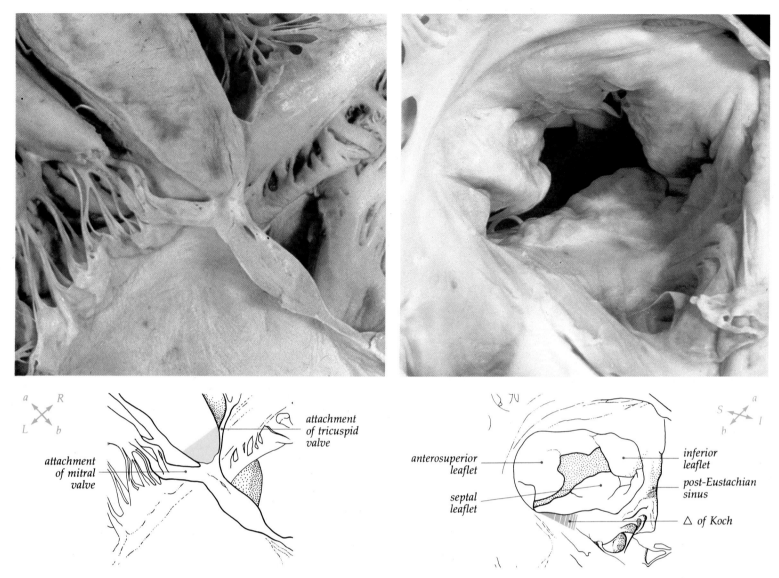

Fig. 2.16 *The more apical insertion of the tricuspid valve relative to the mitral valve creates the atrioventricular muscular septum. This approximates the surgical view were such a section possible.*

Fig. 2.17 *Leaflets of the tricuspid valve and the post-Eustachian sinus in surgical orientation.*

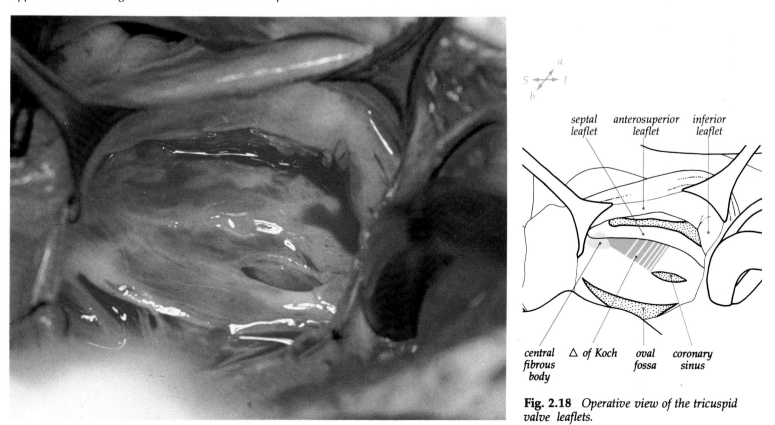

Fig. 2.18 *Operative view of the tricuspid valve leaflets.*

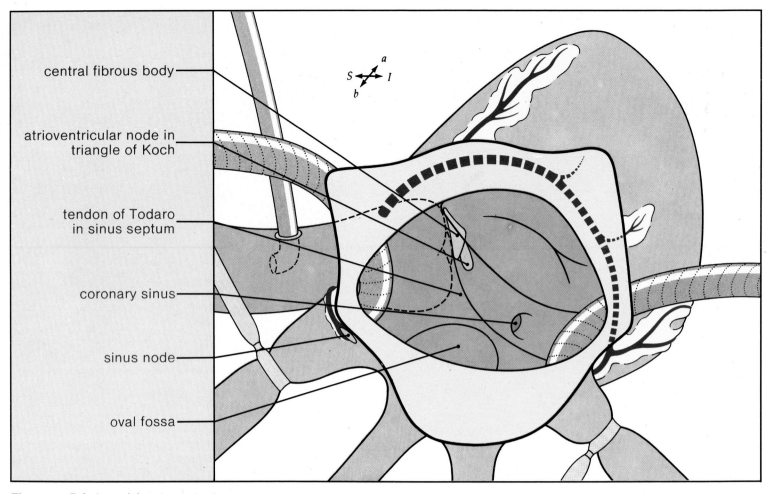

central fibrous body

atrioventricular node in triangle of Koch

tendon of Todaro in sinus septum

coronary sinus

sinus node

oval fossa

Fig. 2.19 *Relations of the tricuspid valve as seen through a right atriotomy. Structures at risk are superimposed. See also Fig. 2.12.*

They are divided from one another by commissures and are tethered by the fan-shaped commissural chordae arising atop the prominent papillary muscles of the valve. Thus the anteroseptal commissure of the tricuspid valve is supported by the medial papillary muscle. This structure is 'around the corner' from the area of the central fibrous body and the membranous septum. The major leaflets of the valve extend from this position in an anterosuperior and septal direction. The third or inferior leaflet of the valve is less well-defined. The anteroinferior commissure is usually supported by the prominent anterior papillary muscle, but this muscle may be attached to only the midpoint of the anterosuperior leaflet. In this case the inferior leaflet may seem to be duplicated, since it is often not possible to identify one specific inferior papillary muscle supporting an inferoseptal commissure. However, this distinction is of minimal surgical significance. The entire parietal attachment of the tricuspid valve is usually encircled by the right coronary artery running in the atrioventricular sulcus (Figs. 2.12 & 2.19). In our experience it is rare to find a well-formed collagenous tricuspid 'annulus'. Instead, the sulcus more or less folds itself directly into the tricuspid valve leaflets and the atrial and ventricular myocardial masses are separated almost exclusively by the adipose tissue of the sulcus.

ii. Morphologically left atrium

Owing to its position, only the appendage of the left atrium may be immediately evident to a surgeon on exposing the heart. As with the right atrium, the left atrium has a venous component in addition to its appendage. However, unlike the right atrium, the venous component of the left atrium is considerably larger than the appendage and the narrow junction of the two parts is unmarked by either a terminal sulcus or crest. Because of its posterior position and its firm anchorage by the four pulmonary veins, the left atrium is relatively inaccessible although there are various routes by which the surgeon may gain access. Probably the most popular route is just posterior to the interatrial groove (Fig. 2.4). As described above, this extensive infolding between the right pulmonary veins and the venous sinus of the right atrium produces the so-called 'secondary septum'. A leftward directed incision along this groove or parallel between it and the right pulmonary veins takes the surgeon directly into the left atrium. If necessary, the incision can be extended to the superior aspect of the left atrium by incising the pericardial fold between the superior caval vein and the right superior pulmonary vein. Because the infolding of the interatrial groove also forms the superior border of the oval fossa, much the same access can be gained

by approaching via the right atrium and incising just superiorly within the fossa. It must then be remembered that an extensive incision may take the surgeon out of the confines of the atria into the pericardial space and may damage the artery to the sinus node. A further approach to the left atrium is the superior approach through the so-called dome. We have already indicated how the crest of the right atrial appendage turns medially into the interatrial groove. If the aorta is pulled anteriorly and to the left, it can be shown that this groove is an extensive trough between the two atrial appendages. An incision through the roof of this trough, between the upper pulmonary veins, provides direct access to the left atrium. However, when making such an incision to enter the left atrium, it must be remembered that the sinus node artery may be coursing upwards through this area from the circumflex artery (45 percent of cases). Also, in some instances this artery may pass through the interatrial groove to reach the terminal sulcus.

When access is gained to the left atrium, the small size of the opening of the appendage is immediately apparent, lying to the left of the mitral orifice as viewed by the surgeon. The greater part of the pulmonary venous atrium will usually be located inferiorly, away from the operative field, and the vestibule of the

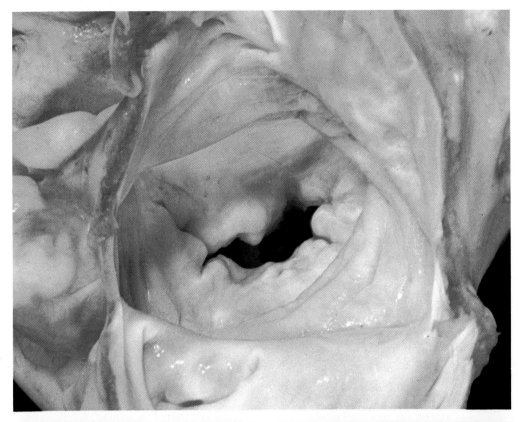

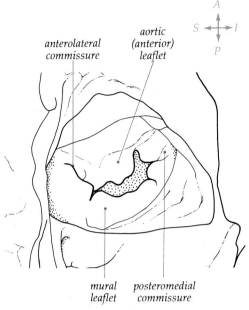

Fig. 2.20 *Leaflets of the mitral valve seen through a left atriotomy parallel to Waterston's groove.*

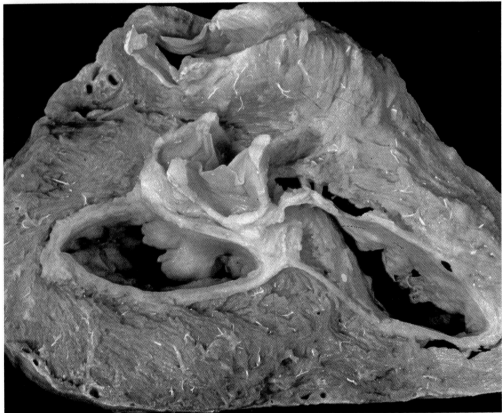

Fig. 2.21 *Cardiac skeleton and coronet-like arrangement of the aortic valve leaflets seen from above and oblique right posteriorly. By courtesy of Prof. A.E. Becker.*

mitral orifice will dominate the picture (Fig. 2.20). The septal aspect will be in a relatively inferior position, exhibiting the typically roughened flap-valve aspect of its left side. The large sweep of tissue between the flap-valve of the septum and the opening of the appendage is the internal aspect of the deep anterior interatrial groove.

The mitral valve is supported by two prominent papillary muscles and their commissural chordae. These are in anterolateral and posteromedial positions.

The two leaflets delineated by these commissures have widely differing appearances (Fig. 2.20). The anterosuperior leaflet is short, squat and relatively square. This is the leaflet in fibrous continuity with the aortic valve and can be termed the aortic leaflet since it is not strictly in either anterior or superior position. The other leaflet is narrower and its annular attachment more extensive, being connected to the parietal part of the mitral annulus. It is accurately termed the mural leaflet and is divided

into a number of subunits by so-called 'cleft chordae'. Usually three in number, it may be possible to find up to five or six of these scallops of the mural leaflet. Unlike the tricuspid valve, the mitral valve leaflets are supported by a rather dense collagenous annulus, usually firmly structured over its circumference, although thinning out in the midportion of its parietal part. The annulus in relation to the aortic leaflet is greatly thickened at each commissure to form the left and right fibrous trigones (Fig. 2.21).

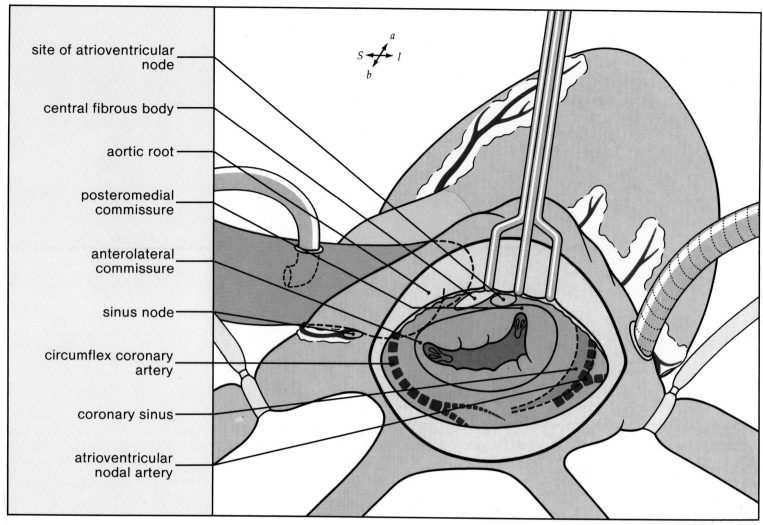

site of atrioventricular node

central fibrous body

aortic root

posteromedial commissure

anterolateral commissure

sinus node

circumflex coronary artery

coronary sinus

atrioventricular nodal artery

Fig. 2.22 *Left atrium opened through an incision parallel to Waterston's groove. The vital related structures have been superimposed.*

The area of the valve orifice and septum related to the right fibrous trigone and central fibrous body is most vulnerable in terms of conduction tissue because here lies the atrioventricular node and penetrating bundle (Fig. 2.22). The area of mitral orifice between the two trigones (more or less the midportion of the aortic leaflet) is directly related to the commissure between the non-coronary and left coronary cusps of the aortic valve. At this point the aortic root is 'tented' up (Fig.

2.21) and an incision apparently through the atrial wall will in fact extend into the subaortic outflow tract. If the incision is continued superiorly the atrial wall will be penetrated into the transverse sinus of the pericardial cavity which overlies the aortic-mitral curtain. The deep inner curvature of the heart overlies and runs to either side of the curtain lined by the transverse sinus. Encircling the mural leaflet of the mitral valve are the circumflex coronary artery from below

and to the left and the coronary sinus from below and to the right (Fig. 2.22). Also, in some cases the atrioventricular nodal artery will run in close proximity to the right side of the mitral orifice, arising from either the circumflex or right coronary artery. The margin directly related to the circumflex artery is somewhat variable; but when the left coronary artery is dominant the entire mural leaflet attachment can be intimately related to the coronary artery (compare Figs. 2.23 & 2.24).

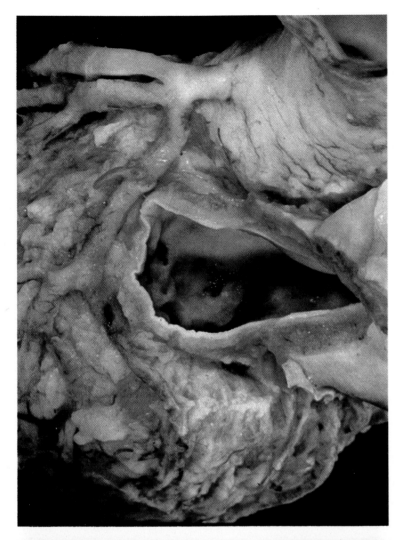

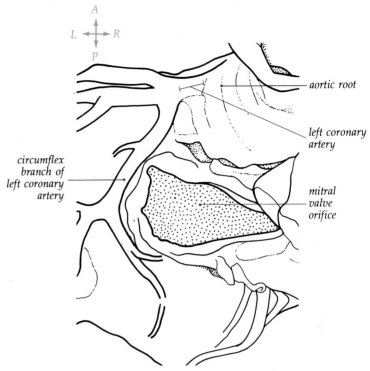

Fig. 2.23 *Relation of a non-dominant left circumflex coronary artery to the mitral valve annulus seen from above and left posteriorly. By courtesy of Prof. A.E. Becker.*

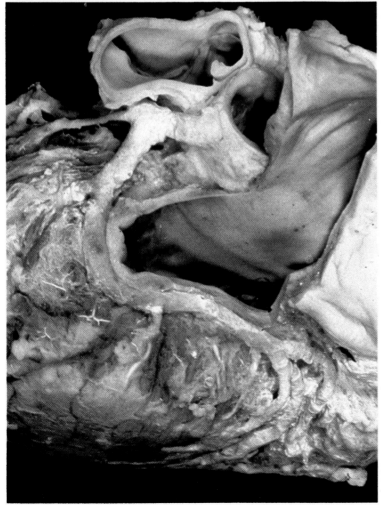

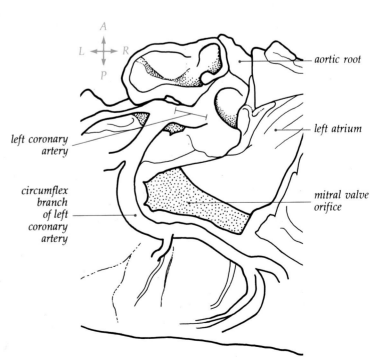

Fig. 2.24 *View as in Fig. 2.23 of a dominant left circumflex artery. By courtesy of Prof. A.E. Becker.*

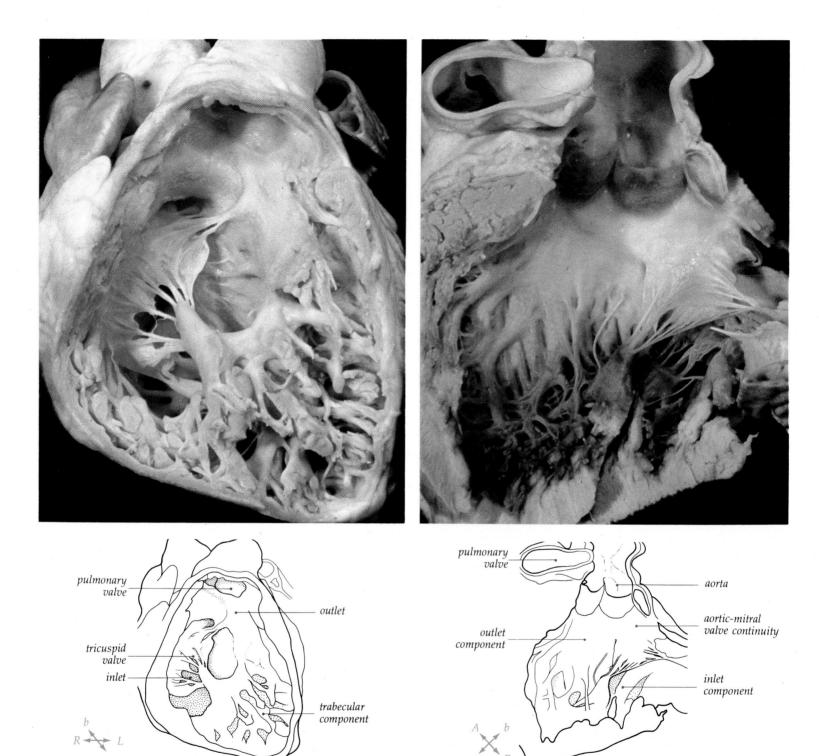

Fig. 2.25 *Right ventricle in anatomical orientation showing the three component parts.*

Fig. 2.26 *Left ventricle in anatomical orientation showing the three component parts by pulling back the parietal wall.*

iii. Morphologically right ventricle

Understanding of both ventricles is greatly aided, in our opinion, by considering their morphology in terms of three components (Figs. 2.25 & 2.26) rather than the traditional 'sinus' and 'conus' parts. The three portions are the inlet, trabecular and outlet parts respectively (*Anderson & Becker, 1980b*). The inlet portion of the right ventricle contains and is limited by the tricuspid valve and its tension apparatus. A distinguishing feature of the tricuspid valve is the direct septal attachments of its septal leaflet. The trabecular component of the right ventricle extends out to the apex, where its wall is particularly thin

and especially vulnerable to perforation by cardiac catheters and pacemaker electrodes. The outlet component of the right ventricle is a complete muscular structure, the infundibulum, which supports the pulmonary valve. The three leaflets of the pulmonary valve do not have an annulus as such; they are attached to the infundibular musculature in semilunar fashion. The pulmonary ring is therefore much higher at the commissures than at the nadir of the leaflet attachments. A distinguishing feature of the right ventricle is the prominent muscular shelf separating the tricuspid and pulmonary valves, the supraventricular crest. Although at first sight (Fig. 2.27) it has

the appearance of a large muscle bundle, much of the crest is no more than the infolded inner heart curve (Fig. 2.28). Incisions or deep sutures through this part would run into the transverse sinus and right atrioventricular groove and would jeopardize the right coronary artery (*McFadden, Culpepper & Ochsner, 1982*). Only the most medial part of the crest is a septal structure, separating the pulmonary valve from the aortic valve (Fig.2.29); it inserts between the limbs of a prominent right ventricular septal trabeculation. This structure, which we term the septomarginal trabecula, has anterior and posterior limbs which clasp the crest.

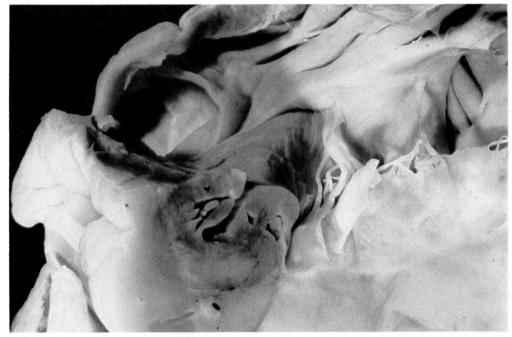

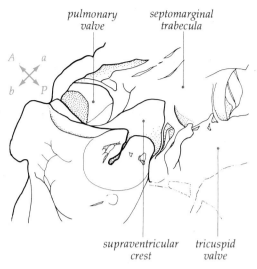

Fig. 2.27 *Normal supraventricular crest inserting between the limbs of the septomarginal trabecula. Surgical orientation. By courtesy of Prof. A.E. Becker.*

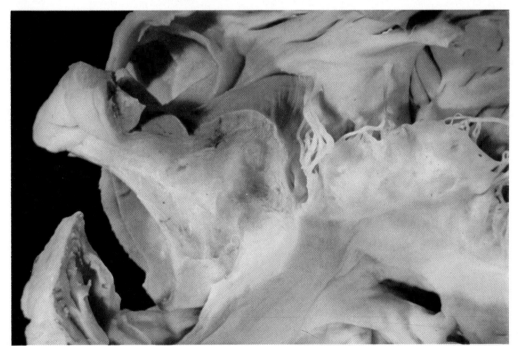

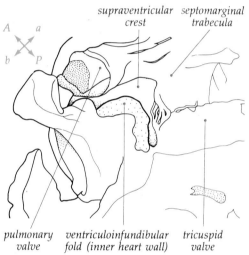

Fig. 2.28 *Most of the crest is made up of the external wall of the heart (the ventriculoinfundibular fold). Surgical orientation. By courtesy of Prof. A.E. Becker.*

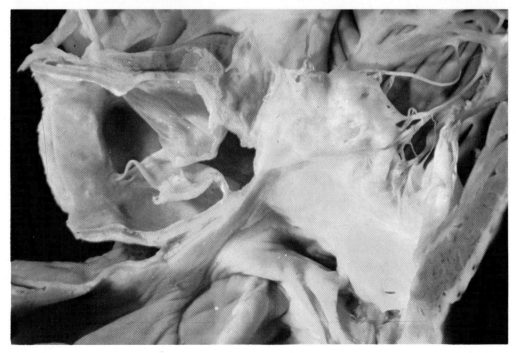

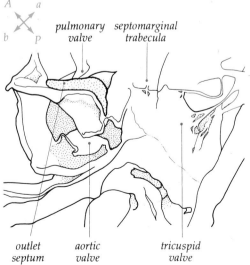

Fig. 2.29 *Only the most medial part of the crest is a septal structure (outlet septum). Surgical orientation. By courtesy of Prof. A.E. Becker.*

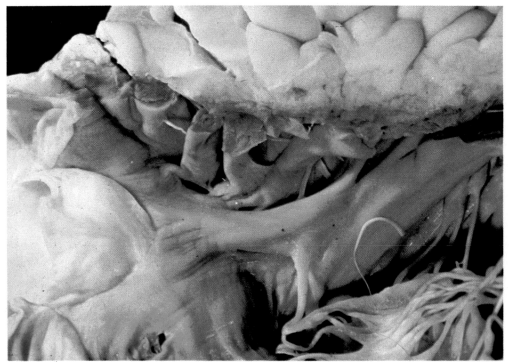

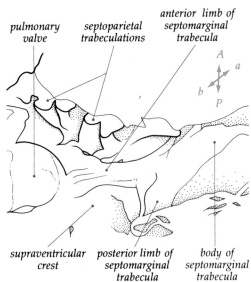

Fig. 2.30 *Septomarginal trabecula and additional septoparietal trabeculations seen in surgical orientation. By courtesy of Prof. A.E. Becker.*

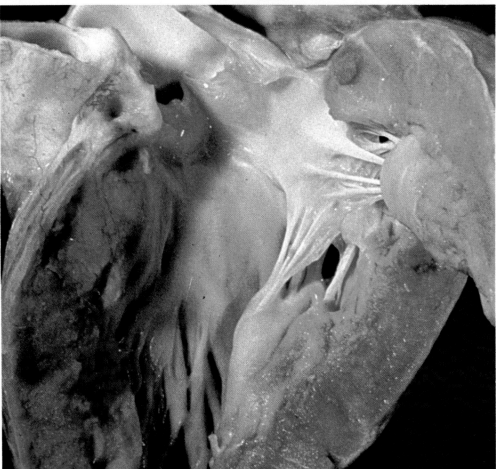

Fig. 2.31 *Posterior diverticulum of the left ventricular outflow tract in anatomical position. The site of the left bundle branch has been superimposed.*

The anterior limb runs up to the pulmonary valve, reinforcing the outlet septum, while the posterior limb extends backwards beneath the interventricular membranous septum to run onto the inlet septum (Fig. 2.30). The medial papillary muscle arises from this posterior limb. The body of the septomarginal trabecula runs to the apex of the ventricle, breaking up into a sheath of smaller trabeculae. Some of these mingle into the trabecular portion and some support tension apparatus of the tricuspid valve. Two trabeculae may be particularly prominent; one becomes the anterior papillary muscle while the other crosses the ventricular cavity and is termed the moderator band. Other significant right ventricular trabeculae are usually found in the trabecular-outlet transitional zone superior and anterior to the septo-marginal trabecula. Variable in number, these are the septoparietal trabeculae (Fig. 2.30).

iv. Morphologically left ventricle

As with the right ventricle, the left ventricle is conveniently considered in terms of inlet, trabecular, and outlet components (Fig. 2.26). The inlet component surrounds and is limited by the mitral valve and its tension apparatus. The papillary muscles of the valve, although basically anterolateral and posteromedial in position, are quite close to each other. Unlike the tricuspid valve, the mitral valve leaflets have no direct

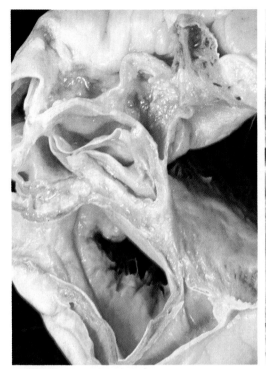

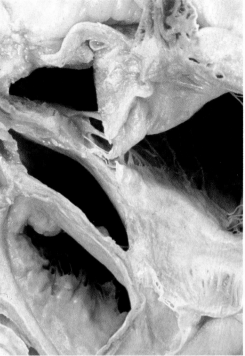

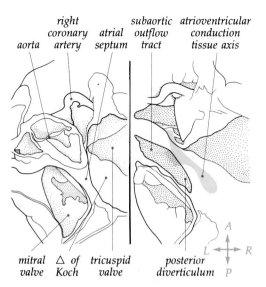

Labels for Fig. 2.32:
aorta · right coronary artery · atrial septum · subaortic outflow tract · atrioventricular conduction tissue axis · mitral valve · △ of Koch · tricuspid valve · posterior diverticulum · A L R P

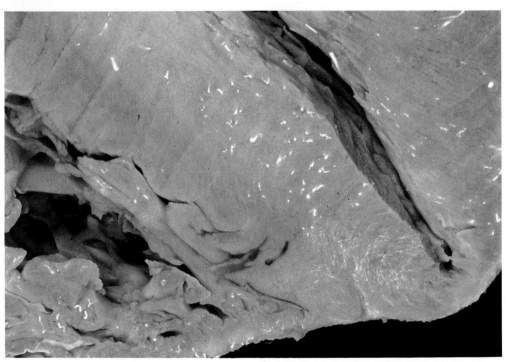

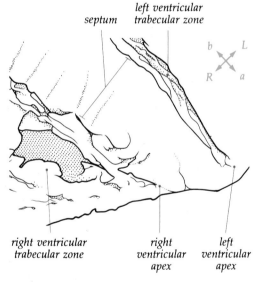

Labels for Fig. 2.33:
septum · left ventricular trabecular zone · right ventricular trabecular zone · right ventricular apex · left ventricular apex · b L R a

Fig. 2.33 *Ventricular walls are very thin at their apices. By courtesy of Prof. A.E. Becker.*

septal attachments (Fig. 2.31), since the deep posterior diverticulum of the outflow tract displaces the aortic leaflet of the mitral valve away from the inlet septum (Fig. 2.32). The trabecular component of the left ventricle extends to the ventricular apex and has characteristically fine trabeculations. As in the right ventricle, the apical myocardium is surprisingly thin (Fig. 2.33). This feature is important to the cardiac surgeon who has reason to place catheters and electrodes in the right ventricle or drainage tubes in the left side. Immediate perforation or delayed rupture may occur. This may be a particular problem with catheters stiffened by hypothermia which are then pushed against the apical endocardium as the heart is manipulated during coronary artery surgery (*Breyer,*

Lavender & Cordell, 1982). The outlet component of the left ventricle supports the aortic valve; but, unlike its right ventricular component, it is not a complete muscular structure. The septal wall is largely composed of muscle, but the membranous septum forms part of the subaortic outflow tract. The deep posterior diverticulum of the outflow tract is that space extending from the septum across to the aortic leaflet of the mitral valve. The left lateral quadrant round to the septum is then a muscular structure, the lateral margin of the inner heart curvature lined by transverse sinus. The muscular septal surface of the outflow tract is characteristically smooth and down this surface cascades the fan-like left bundle branch. The landmark of the descent of the left bundle branch is the

membranous septum immediately beneath the commissure between right coronary and non-coronary cusps of the aortic valve (Fig. 2.31). The left bundle descends initially as a relatively narrow solitary fascicle but soon divides into three interconnected fascicles which radiate into anterior, septal and posterior positions. The interconnecting radiations do not fan out to any degree until the bundle itself has descended to between one-third and one-half the length of the septum. As with the pulmonary valve, the aortic valve does not have an annulus as such, since the leaflets are attached in semilunar fashion. Because this valve forms the keystone of the heart and because it is related to each of the other cardiac chambers and valves, we will describe its morphology in more detail.

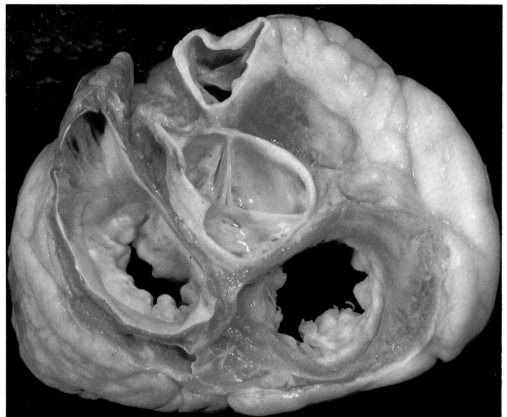

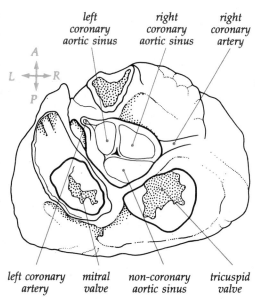

left coronary aortic sinus | right coronary aortic sinus | right coronary artery

left coronary artery | mitral valve | non-coronary aortic sinus | tricuspid valve

Fig. 2.34 *Short-axis view from above of the wedged position of the aortic valve.*

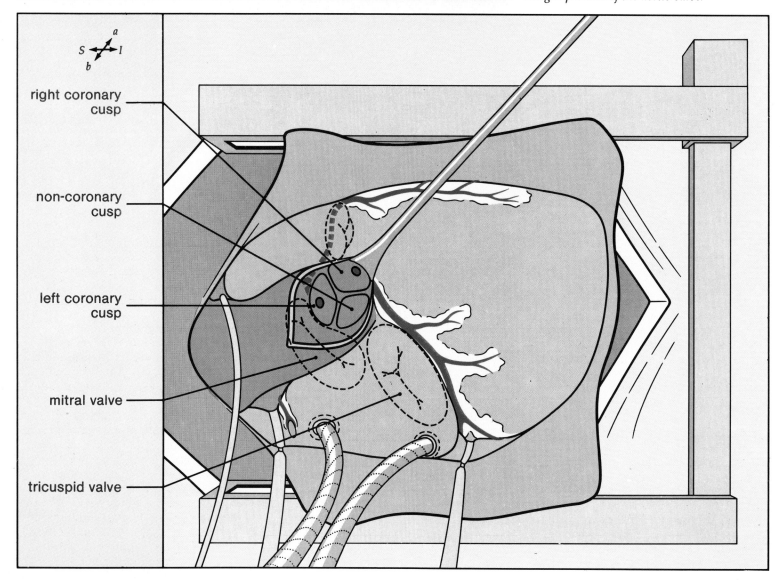

right coronary cusp

non-coronary cusp

left coronary cusp

mitral valve

tricuspid valve

Fig. 2.35 *Important relationships of the aortic valve in surgical orientation.*

2.18

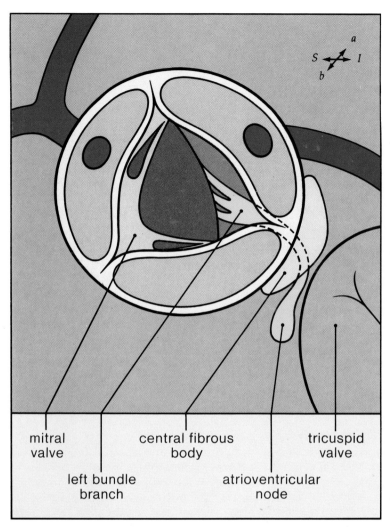

Fig. 2.36 *Relations of the aortic valve as seen through an aortotomy.*

mitral
valve

central fibrous
body

tricuspid
valve

left bundle
branch

atrioventricular
node

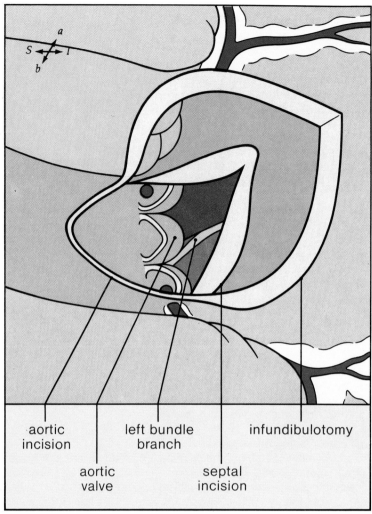

Fig. 2.37 *Approach to the left ventricular outflow tract through the infundibulum of the right ventricle in surgical orientation.*

aortic
incision

left bundle
branch

infundibulotomy

aortic
valve

septal
incision

v. The aortic valve

The subaortic outflow tract has muscular and fibrous parts; therefore, the three semilunar leaflets, or cusps, of the aortic valve have in part fibrous and in part muscular attachments. The leaflets themselves are attached within the expanded aortic sinuses. Because two of these sinuses give rise to coronary arteries and one does not, the aortic leaflets can conveniently be named after their sinuses as the right coronary, left coronary and non-coronary leaflets (Fig. 2.34). However, because of the oblique position of the aortic root, the sinuses themselves are rarely in strictly right and left position (see below). When the aortic wall is removed, the attachments of the valve can be seen to be in the form of a three-piece coronet, with the three commissures forming its highest points (Fig. 2.21). The commissure between the non-coronary

and left coronary leaflets is positioned along the area of aortic-mitral valve continuity. Beneath this commissure is the so-called fibrous subaortic curtain. To the right relative to this commissure, the non-coronary leaflet is attached above the extensive posterior diverticulum of the outflow tract. This is the part of the valve directly related to the right atrial wall (Figs. 2.34 & 2.35). From the inferior attachment of the non-coronary leaflet in relation to the right atrium, the valve tents up again to the commissure between the non-coronary and right coronary leaflets. The ascending part of the non-coronary leaflet is then positioned directly above the part of the atrial septum containing the atrioventricular node, while the commissure itself is above the penetrating atrioventricular bundle and the membranous septum (Fig. 2.36). The

commissure between the right coronary and left coronary leaflets is usually positioned opposite a facing commissure of the pulmonary valve. Therefore, the adjacent parts of these two coronary leaflets are attached to the outlet part of the ventricular septum and are thus directly related to the infundibulum of the right ventricle. Indeed, incisions through the right ventricular outflow tract at this site lead directly into the subaortic region (Fig. 2.37). This is the basis of the right ventricular approach for relief of subaortic obstruction. Beyond this point, the lateral part of the left coronary leaflet is the only part of the aortic valve not intimately related to another cardiac chamber. This is the part of the valve which takes origin from the lateral margin of the inner heart curvature and is, therefore, in relationship externally with the free pericardial space.

vi. The aorta

The ascending aorta begins at the aortic bar, which lies just at the opening line of the free edge of the aortic valve cusps. It runs its short course passing superiorly, obliquely to the right and slightly forward toward the sternum. It is contained within the fibrous pericardium so its surface is covered with serous pericardium. Its anterior surface abuts directly on the pulmonary trunk which is otherwise also covered with serous pericardium. The two vessels together make up the so-called vascular pedicle leading from the heart. The ascending aorta is related anteriorly to the right atrial appendage, the right ventricular outflow tract and pulmonary trunk. Extrapericardially the thymus gland lies between it and the sternum. The medial wall of the right atrium, the superior caval vein and the right pleura relate to its right side. On the left its principal relationship is with the pulmonary trunk. Posterior to the ascending aorta lies the transverse sinus of the pericardium (see above) separating it from the left atrium and right pulmonary artery.

The arch of the aorta begins at the superior attachment of the pericardial reflection just proximal to the origin of the brachiocephalic (innominate) artery. It continues superiorly briefly before coursing posteriorly and to the left, crossing the lateral aspect of the distal trachea and finally terminating on the lateral aspect of the vertebral column. Here it is 'tethered' by the parietal pleura and the arterial ligament. During its course, it gives off the brachiocephalic, the left common carotid and the left subclavian arteries. Bronchial arteries may arise from the arch and can be particularly troublesome if not carefully identified in patients with coarctation of the aorta. The left phrenic and vagus nerves run over the anterolateral aspect of the arch just beneath the mediastinal pleura. The left recurrent laryngeal nerve branches from the vagus to curl superiorly around the arterial ligament before passing on to the posterior medial side of the arch. Here the arch relates to the tracheal bifurcation and oesophagus on its medial border but also to the left main bronchus and pulmonary artery inferiorly (Fig. 2.38).

The descending or thoracic aorta continues from the arch, running a course lateral to the vertebral bodies initially and reaching an anterior position at its termination. Throughout its course it gives off many branches to the viscera of the thorax as well as to the prominent lower nine pairs of intercostal arteries. These latter vessels are of critical concern for the cardiac surgeon. In coarctation of the aorta they serve as primary collateral vessels to bypass the obstructed aorta, accounting for the rib notching seen in older children with coarctation. These vessels and branches to the chest wall can

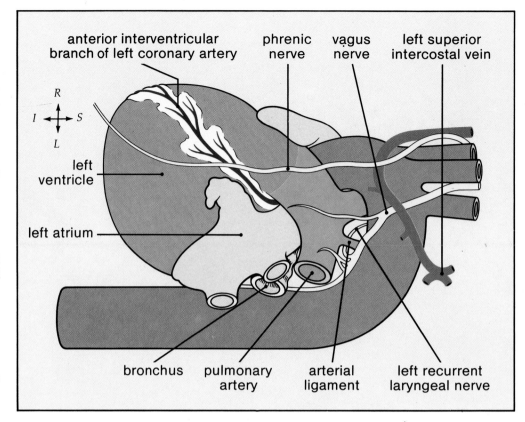

Fig. 2.38 *Relations of the aortic arch viewed from the left thoracic cavity.*

be a source of troublesome bleeding if not properly secured when operating on such patients. Also, the surgeon must remember that the dorsal branches of the intercostal vessels contribute a spinal branch which is important in the blood supply to the spinal cord. Because it is difficult to predict exactly where these vital branches will arise the surgeon must make every attempt to protect the origin of these intercostal vessels from permanent occlusion.

vii. The pulmonary arteries

The pulmonary trunk is a short vessel, usually less than five centimetres in length in the adult. It is completely contained within the pericardium and, similar to its running mate, the ascending aorta, is covered with a layer of serous pericardium except where the two vessels abut each other in the vascular pedicle. It takes origin from the most anterior aspect of the heart, lying just behind the lateral edge of the sternum and the second left intercostal space. Initially the pulmonary trunk overlies the aorta and left coronary artery, but it soon moves to a side by side position with the ascending aorta. The left

coronary artery turns abruptly anteriorly to lie between the left atrial appendage and the pulmonary trunk. The arterial ligament extends from the aorta to the very end of the pulmonary trunk as the latter divides into left and right pulmonary arteries. The left pulmonary artery courses laterally in front of the descending aorta and left main stem bronchus before it sends branches to the hilum of the lung. Posteroinferiorly the left pulmonary artery is connected to the left superior pulmonary vein by a fold of serous pericardium containing a ligamentous remnant of the left superior caval vein, the ligament of Marshall. The right pulmonary artery is somewhat longer than the left, having to traverse the mediastinum through the aortic arch and then behind the superior caval vein. It lies in a posteroinferior position relative to the azygos vein and is anterior to the left main bronchus. The right pulmonary artery often branches before reaching the lateral wall of the superior caval vein while still posterior to the transverse sinus of the pericardium. Thus, a large upper lobar branch may be mistaken for the main right pulmonary artery.

Anderson, K.R., Ho, S.Y. & Anderson, R.H. (1979) The location and vascular supply of the sinus node in the human heart. *British Heart Journal*, **41**, 28–32.

Anderson, R.H. & Becker, A.E. (1980a) *Cardiac Anatomy. An Integrated Text and Colour Atlas*, pp 2.19–2.21. London, Edinburgh: Gower Medical Publishing — Churchill Livingstone.

Anderson, R.H. & Becker, A.E. (1980b) *Cardiac Anatomy. An Integrated Text and Colour Atlas*, pp 3.2–3.3. London, Edinburgh: Gower Medical Publishing — Churchill Livingstone.

Anderson, R.H., Ho, S.Y., Smith, A. & Becker, A.E. (1981) The internodal atrial myocardium. *Anatomical Record*, **201**, 75–82.

Anderson, R.H., Smith, A. & Wilkinson, J.L. (1976) Right juxtaposition of the auricular appendages. *European*

Journal of Cardiology, **4**, 495–503.

Breyer, R.H., Lavender, S. & Cordell, A.R. (1982) Delayed left ventricular rupture secondary to transatrial left ventricular vent. *Annals of Thoracic Surgery*, **33**, 189–191.

James, T.N. (1961) *Anatomy of Coronary Arteries.* New York: Hoeber.

McFadden, P.M., Culpepper, W.S. & Ochsner, J.L. (1982) Iatrogenic right ventricular failure in tetralogy of Fallot repairs: reappraisal of a distressing problem. *Annals of Thoracic Surgery*, **33**, 400–402.

Melhuish, B.P.P. & Van Praagh, R. (1968) Juxtaposition of the atrial appendages. A sign of severe cyanotic congenital heart disease. *British Heart Journal*, **30**, 269–284.

Sweeney, L.J. & Rosenquist, G.C. (1979) The normal anatomy of the atrial septum in the human heart. *American Heart Journal*, **98**, 194–199.

3 Surgical Anatomy of the Coronary Circulation

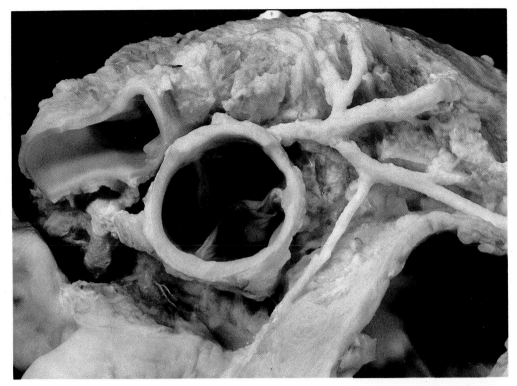

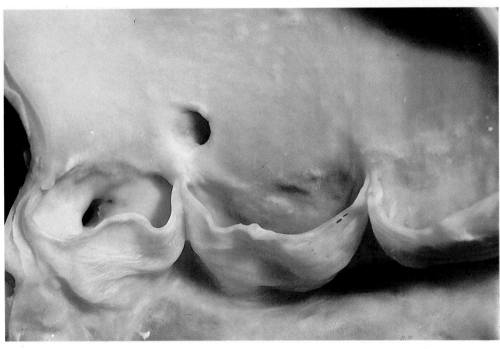

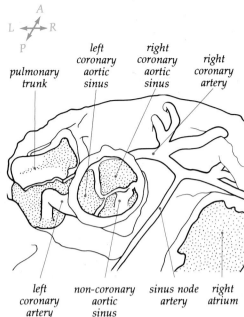

Fig. 3.1 *Origin of the coronary arteries from the aortic sinuses which face the pulmonary trunk.*

Fig. 3.2 *Opened aortic root in anatomical orientation viewed from the left posterior aspect showing origin of the right coronary artery above the aortic bar. By courtesy of Prof. A.E. Becker.*

The coronary circulation comprises the coronary arteries, the coronary veins and the lymphatics of the heart. The lymphatics are of very limited significance to operative anatomy and will not be discussed further. The veins are also of little interest, so this chapter is concentrated upon the anatomic aspects of arterial distribution which are pertinent to the surgeon.

The coronary arteries are the first branches of the ascending portion of the aorta and arise from the aortic root immediately above its attachment to the heart. Normally, there are three aortic sinuses at the aortic root but only two coronary arteries. The sinuses are therefore named according to whether or not they give rise to an artery, the normal arrangement being a right coronary, left coronary and non-coronary sinus (Fig. 3.1). The terms 'right' and 'left' coronary sinuses are not strictly accurate because of the oblique position of the aortic root in the normal heart. Furthermore, in malformed hearts the aortic root is frequently abnormally situated. However, whatever the position of the aortic root, almost always the two coronary arteries (when two are present) take origin from the aortic sinuses which face the pulmonary trunk. Therefore it is more convenient, and more accurate, to term these sinuses the left- and right-facing sinuses.

The coronary arteries arise from the aortic sinuses immediately beneath the transition zone between the aortic root and the tubular ascending aorta (the aortic bar). The free edge of the aortic valve leaflets usually opens against this bar during ventricular systole. Deviations of origin of the coronary arteries relative to the aortic bar are not uncommon (*Neufeld & Schneeweiss, 1983*) and, indeed, are considered abnormal only when they arise more than one centimetre from the bar. According to Bader (1963), this occurs in 3.5 percent of hearts. The arterial opening can be deviated either towards the aortic origin so that the artery arises deep within the aortic sinus, or towards the aortic arch so that arterial origin is outside the sinus (Fig. 3.2). Such displacement may lead to the artery taking an oblique course through the aortic wall, which introduces the potential for luminal narrowing and myocardial perfusion disturbances, particularly when the deviated origin is intimately related to a

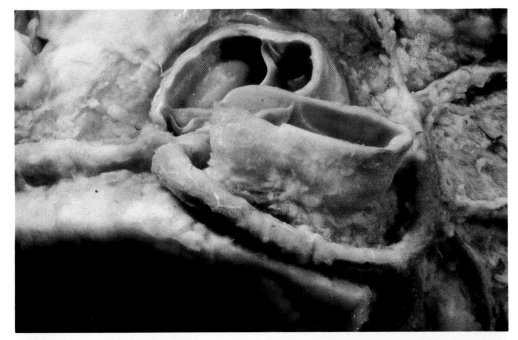

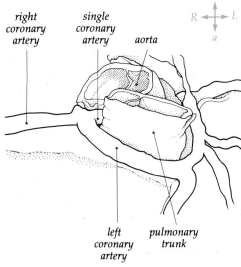

right coronary artery   single coronary artery   aorta

left coronary artery   pulmonary trunk

Fig. 3.3 *Single coronary artery seen in anatomical orientation. By courtesy of Prof. A.E. Becker.*

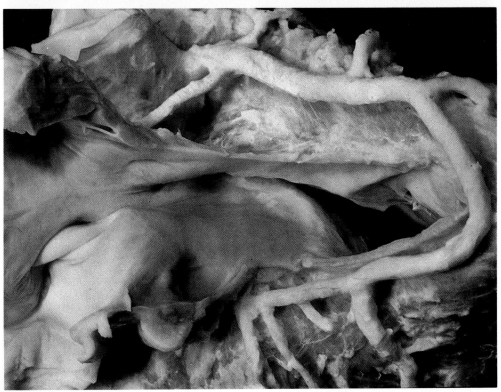

aorta   right coronary artery   acute marginal branch

right atrium   right atrioventricular groove   tricuspid valve orifice

Fig. 3.4 *Tricuspid orifice viewed obliquely from the right and above showing its intimate relationship to the right coronary artery.*

valve commissure (*Becker, 1981*).

The left coronary artery almost always takes origin from a single orifice. On the other hand, in about half of all hearts there are two coronary orifices within the right-facing sinus. These orifices are unequal in size; the larger gives rise to the main trunk of the right coronary artery, while the considerably smaller second orifice usually gives rise to an infundibular artery. In the series reported by Becker (1981), two orifices were found in 46 percent of cases, three orifices in 7 percent and four orifices in 2 percent. These multiple right coronary orifices are of little surgical significance. In contrast, multiple left orifices, although considerably more rare (found in only eight of the 4250 patients reported by Engel, Torres and Page, 1975), do have

clinical significance. Unless recognized, they can create problems in the interpretation of coronary angiograms.

The coronary arteries can also arise, though rarely, from a single coronary orifice, usually within the right-facing sinus. The single artery produces one of two patterns. In the first, the single artery immediately divides into right and left coronary arteries (Fig. 3.3), with the left artery passing either in front of or behind the pulmonary trunk before dividing into anterior interventricular (descending) and circumflex branches. In the second and rarer pattern, the single artery follows the path of the normal right coronary artery and continues beyond the crux, encircling the mitral orifice to terminate as the anterior interventricular coronary artery.

The epicardial course of the major

coronary arteries follows the atrioventricular and interventricular grooves. The right coronary artery emerges from the right-facing aortic sinus and immediately enters the right atrioventricular groove. It then encircles the tricuspid orifice within the fat pad of the groove (Fig. 3.4). In approximately nine-tenths of cases, the right coronary artery gives rise to a posterior interventricular artery at the crux (dominant right coronary artery). In a good proportion of these the artery continues beyond the crux and supplies downgoing branches to the diaphragmatic surface of the left ventricle. As the right coronary encircles the tricuspid orifice, it is most closely related to the annulus near the acute margin and the origin of its acute marginal branch.

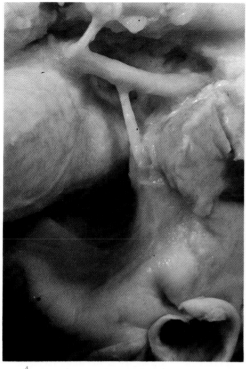

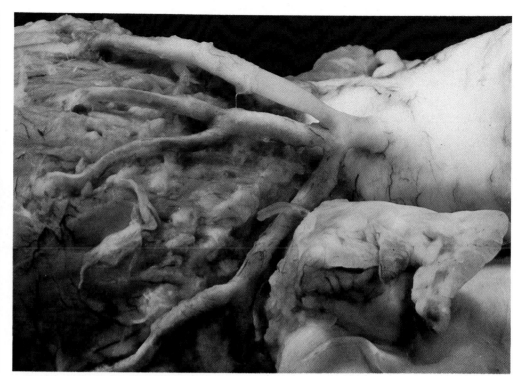

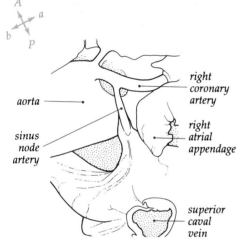

Fig. 3.5 *Origin of the sinus node artery from the right coronary artery.*

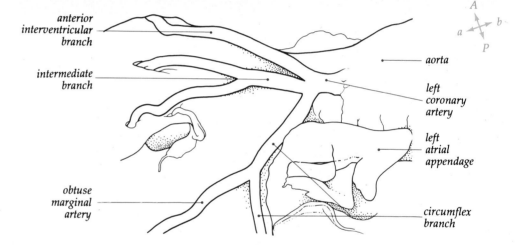

Fig. 3.6 *An intermediate branch of the left coronary artery viewed laterally from the left.*

The right coronary artery also gives off other important branches in its encircling segment. Immediately after its origin the artery is within the ventriculoinfundibular fold, where it gives rise to downgoing infundibular branches (which may also arise by separate orifices; see above). In just over half the cases it gives rise to the sinus node artery (Fig. 3.5).

The left main coronary artery emerges from the left-facing sinus into the left margin of the ventriculoinfundibular fold behind the pulmonary trunk and beneath the left atrial appendage. It is a very short structure, rarely extending beyond one centimetre before branching into the anterior interventricular and circumflex branches. In some hearts the main stem trifurcates with an intermediate branch between the other main branches (Fig. 3.6). The intermediate branch supplies the pulmonary surface (obtuse margin) of the left ventricle. The anterior interventricular artery runs down the anterior interventricular groove, giving off

diagonal branches to the obtuse margin and the important perforating branches which pass posteriorly into the septum. The artery then continues towards the apex and frequently curves under the apex to pass onto the diaphragmatic surface. The circumflex branch of the left coronary artery passes backwards to run in close relationship with the mitral orifice. It is most closely related to the orifice when it gives rise to the posterior interventricular artery at the crux (dominant left coronary artery; Fig. 3.7). A dominant left coronary artery is found in only about one-tenth of cases. When the left coronary is not dominant, the circumflex artery usually terminates by supplying downgoing branches to the pulmonary surface of the left ventricle.

Throughout much of their epicardial course the arteries and their accompanying veins are encased in epicardial adipose tissue. In some hearts the myocardium itself may form a 'bridge' over segments of the artery. The role of

these 'bridges' in the development of coronary arterial disease is not clear; certainly they can be an impediment to the surgeon in his effort to isolate the artery for bypass.

The importance of knowing the precise course of the sinus node artery when deciding how to approach the different cardiac chambers has already been discussed in Chapter 2, where we illustrated the right lateral sinus node artery (see Fig. 2.9). This variant, rare in normal hearts, was discovered in three of 27 hearts we have dissected with congenital malformations (Fig. 3.8). Of equal significance was our finding that whenever the nodal artery coursed retrocavally it burrowed deep within the interatrial (Waterston's) groove (Fig. 3.9). In this position it could be at risk in the operative approach to the mitral valve through the groove or in operations which mobilize the tissues of the groove, such as the Senning procedure.

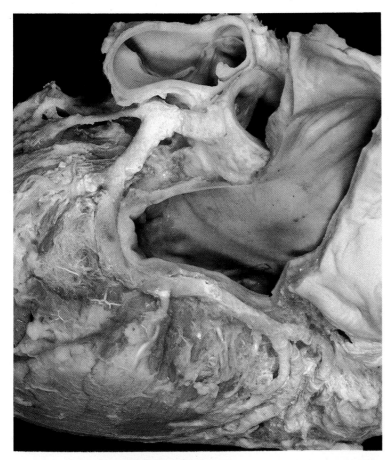

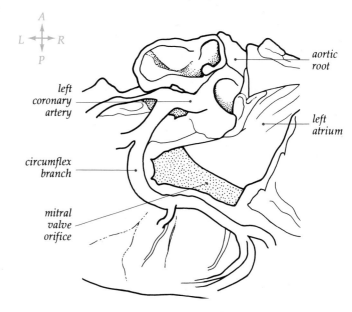

Fig. 3.7 *The intimate relationship of a dominant left coronary artery to the mitral valve ring.*

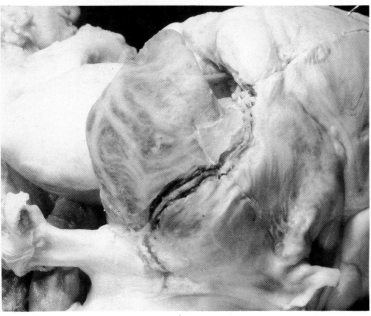

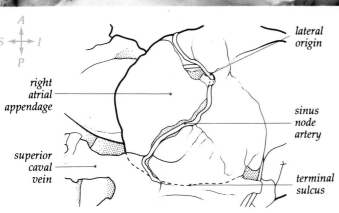

Fig. 3.8 *Right sinus node artery with lateral origin as seen in an autopsied case of tetralogy of Fallot. By courtesy of Dr. J. Busquet, University of Bordeaux.*

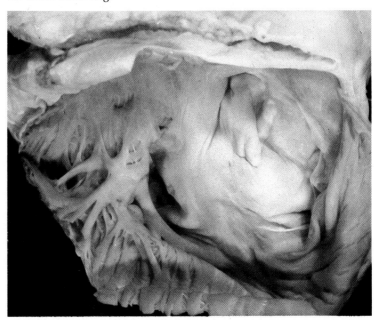

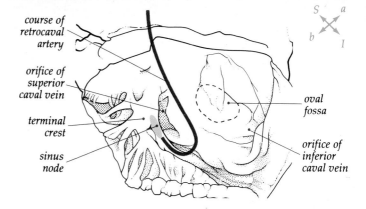

Fig. 3.9 *Opened right atrium with retrocaval sinus node artery. The position of the artery relative to the oval fossa and terminal crest has been superimposed.*

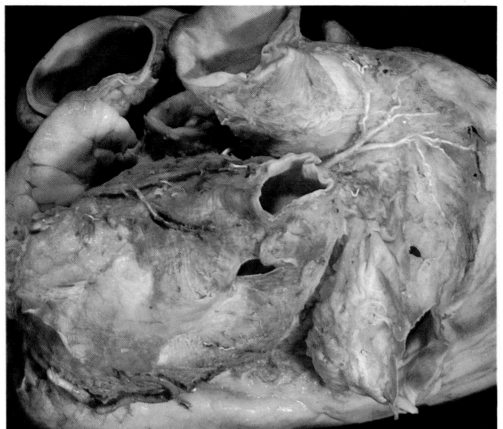

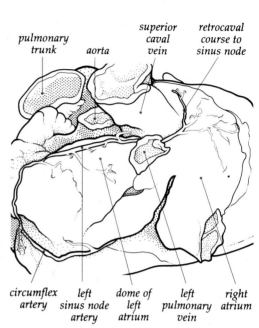

pulmonary trunk   aorta   superior caval vein   retrocaval course to sinus node

circumflex artery   left sinus node artery   dome of left atrium   left pulmonary vein   right atrium

Fig. 3.10 *Course of a left sinus node artery across the dome of the left atrium.*

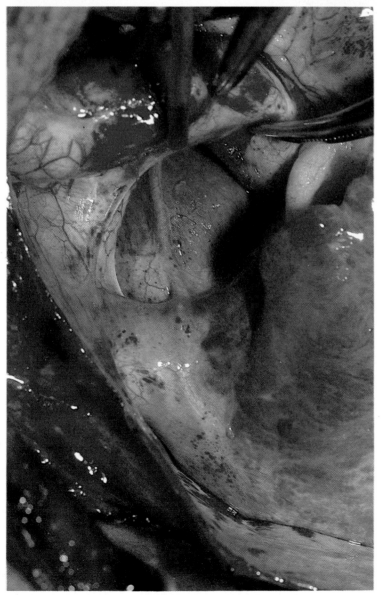

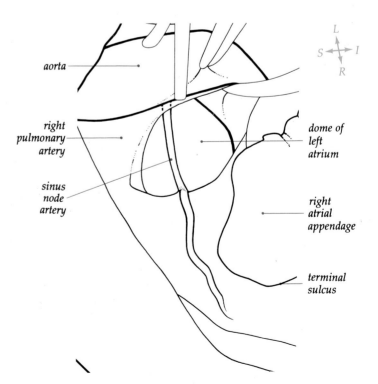

aorta

right pulmonary artery   dome of left atrium

sinus node artery

right atrial appendage

terminal sulcus

Fig. 3.11 *Course of a left sinus node artery across the dome of the left atrium seen at operation.*

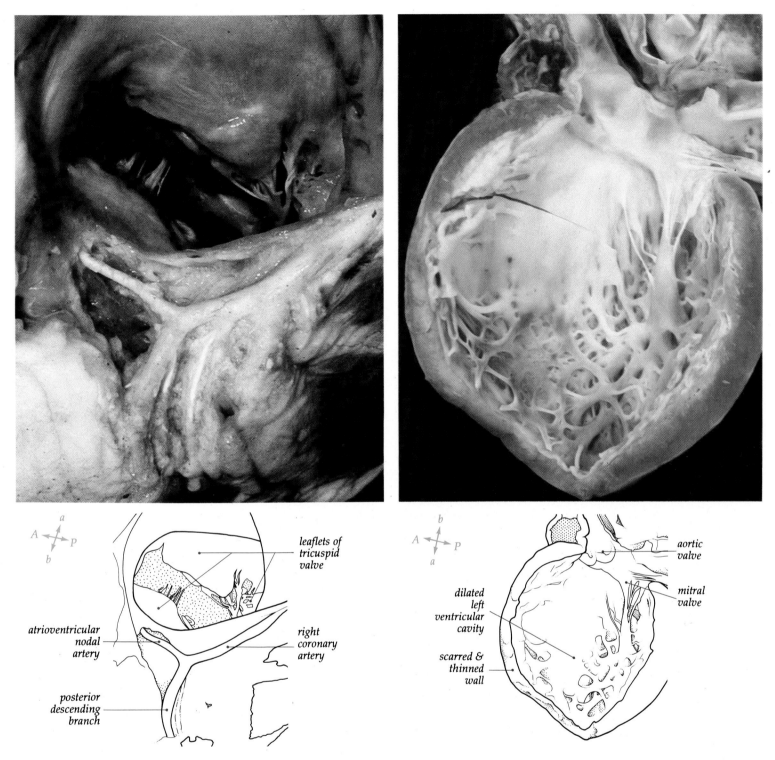

Fig. 3.12 *Origin of the atrioventricular nodal artery from the dominant right coronary artery in surgical orientation. By courtesy of Prof. A.E. Becker.*

Fig. 3.13 *Dilated left ventricle with a thinned and scarred wall due to ischaemia because of anomalous origin of the left coronary artery from the pulmonary trunk.*

We have also observed, both in dissections (Fig. 3.10) and at operation (Fig. 3.11), the arrangement in which a left sinus node artery courses across the dome of the atrium. An approach to the mitral valve or left atrium through the dome would put this artery at risk. All in all, the sinus node artery may be at risk in a significant number of cases (*Busquet et al., 1984*).

The arterial supply to the ventricular conduction tissues is also of surgical significance. The atrioventricular nodal artery arises from the dominant coronary artery at the crux, usually from a U-turn of

this artery beneath the floor of the coronary sinus. The nodal artery then passes towards the central fibrous body, running into the fibrofatty plane of the atrioventricular groove (Fig. 3.12) to enter the node. In some hearts it then perforates the fibrous annulus to supply a good part of the branching atrioventricular bundle. The septal perforating arteries from the anterior interventricular artery always supply the anterior parts of the ventricular bundle branches and, occasionally, also supply the greater part of the posterior ventricular conduction tissues (*Anderson & Becker, 1980*).

Thus far we have considered the surgical significance of anomalous origins of the coronary arteries from the aortic root. There are other congenital malformations of the coronary arteries which, although rare, require consideration. The most important of these is origin of one coronary artery from the pulmonary trunk, particularly when it is a left coronary artery. This lesion produces ischaemia of the left ventricle, which can progress to infarction with or without mitral insufficiency (Fig. 3.13). Another feature is the development of extensive collateral communications with the right

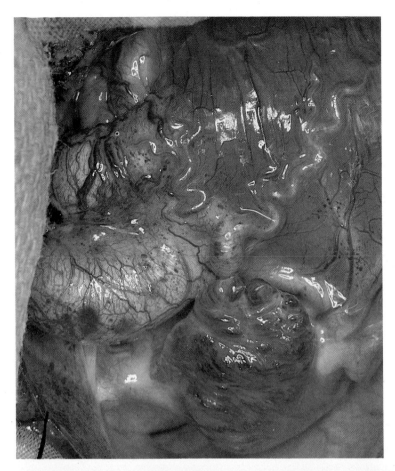

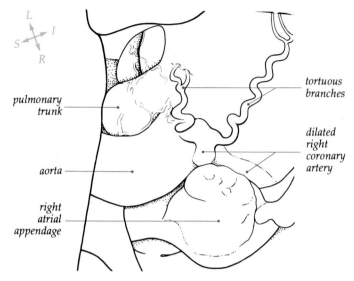

Fig. 3.14 *Operative view of a large tortuous right coronary artery associated with anomalous origin of the left coronary artery from the pulmonary trunk.*

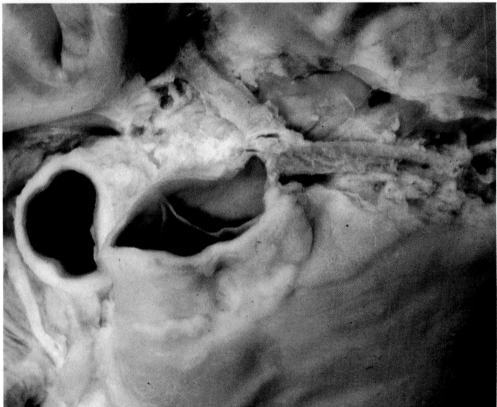

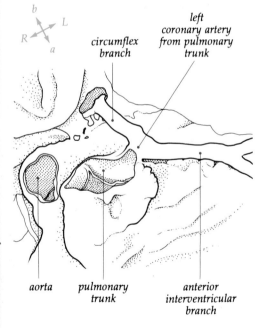

Fig. 3.15 *Anomalous origin of the left coronary artery from the pulmonary trunk. By courtesy of Prof. A.E. Becker.*

coronary artery (Fig. 3.14). These may permit a 'steal' situation with flow from the right coronary artery to the left and thence to the pulmonary trunk. Although the anomalous artery usually arises from the left-facing pulmonary sinus, it is still some distance from the aorta (Fig. 3.15).

This may make transplantation or construction of an aortopulmonary

fenestration difficult. An alternative procedure is detachment of the artery from the pulmonary trunk and anastomosis to a systemic artery such as the subclavian. Simple ligation has also been advocated when the collateral circulation is well developed. Exceedingly rarely, both coronary arteries may arise from the pulmonary trunk (*Keeton, Keenan & Monro, 1983*). Unless recognized

immediately and treated surgically, this anomaly is incompatible with life.

Another congenital coronary arterial malformation of considerable clinical significance is abnormal communications between the coronary arteries and either the cardiac chambers or the cardiac veins. Coronary-cameral fistulae, excluding those present in cases with valve atresia, are rare. Rittenhouse, Doty and Ehrenhaft

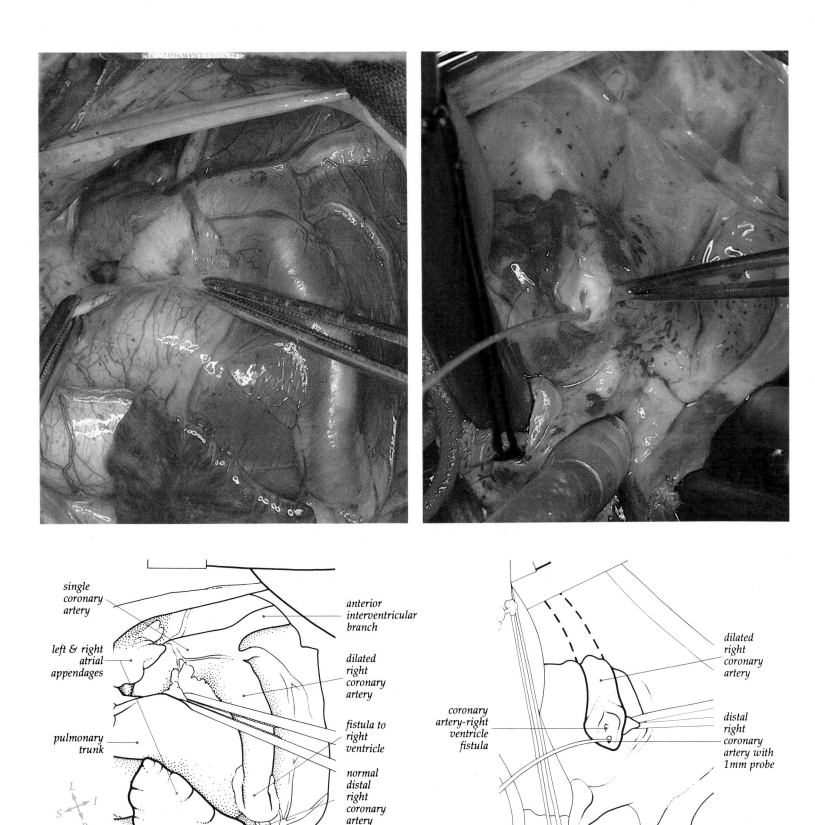

Fig. 3.16 *Operative views of a fistula between the right coronary artery and the right ventricle. The single coronary artery gives rise to a grossly dilated right coronary artery (left) which becomes normal beyond the site of the fistulous communication (right).*

(1975) reported on 163 patients, gathered from the English literature, who had undergone surgical treatment. They showed that the right coronary artery was most frequently involved and the fistulae most often terminated in the right ventricle (Fig. 3.16). However, the left coronary artery was involved in 41 percent of cases and, in 8 percent, both arteries contributed to the fistula. These fistulae can drain into any of the cardiac chambers or into the superior caval vein, coronary sinus, pulmonary artery or pulmonary vein. The involved artery is quite dilated and runs a tortuous course. In most cases the surgical treatment is simple ligation of the fistula, though cardiopulmonary bypass may be required. In advocating the use of cardiopulmonary bypass, Horiuchi and his associates (1971) pointed out the potential hazard of proximal ligation of a right coronary arterial fistula communicating with the right atrium or superior caval vein, in other words, injury to the atrioventricular nodal artery. A significant feature of this particular anomaly is the relatively low incidence of associated congenital cardiac malformations.

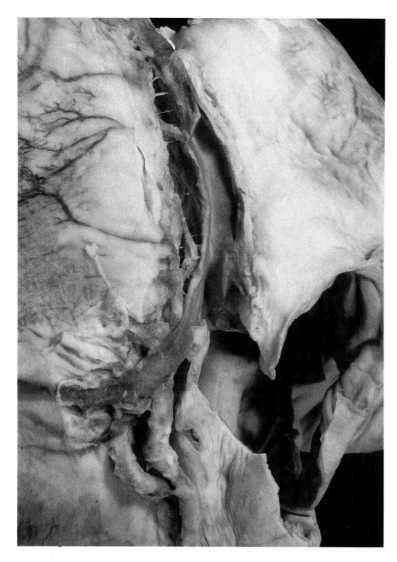

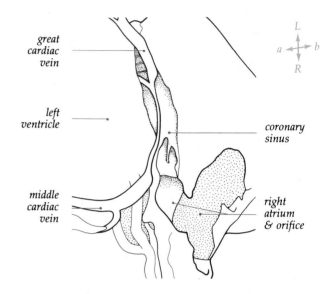

great cardiac vein

left ventricle

middle cardiac vein

coronary sinus

right atrium & orifice

Fig. 3.17 *Coronary veins drain into the coronary sinus which in turn terminates in the right atrium.*

There are other congenital anomalies of the heart where abnormal dispositions of the coronary arteries constitute an important feature of the surgical anatomy. These will be dealt with in their own sections.

The coronary veins drain blood from the myocardium to the right atrium. The smaller veins (anterior and smallest cardiac veins) which drain directly to the cavity of the atrium are not of surgical significance. The larger veins accompany the major arteries and run into the coronary sinus (Fig. 3.17). The great cardiac vein runs alongside the anterior interventricular artery and becomes the coronary sinus as it encircles the mitral orifice to enter the posterior left margin of the atrioventricular groove. The coronary sinus then runs along the groove, lying between the left atrial wall and the ventricular myocardium, before draining into the right atrium between the sinus septum and the post-Eustachian sinus. At the crux the coronary sinus receives the middle cardiac vein, which has ascended with the posterior interventricular artery, and the small cardiac vein, which has encircled the tricuspid orifice in company with the right coronary artery. Occasionally, these latter two veins drain directly to the right atrium. The orifice of the coronary sinus is guarded by the Thebesian valve, which may be imperforate. Other valves are found within the cardiac veins; that found in the great cardiac vein where it turns round the pulmonary surface is called the valve of Vieussens.

Anderson, R.H. & Becker, A.E. (1980) *Cardiac Anatomy. An Integrated Text and Colour Atlas*, pp 6.28–6.29. London, Edinburgh: Gower Medical Publishing-Churchill Livingstone.
Bader, G. (1963) Beitrag zur Systematik und Haufigkeit der Anomalien der Coronararterien des Menschen. *Virchow Archives of Pathology and Anatomy*, **337**, 88–96.
Becker, A.E. (1981) Variations of the main coronary arteries. In *Paediatric Cardiology Volume 3*, pp 263–277. Edited by A.E. Becker, G. Losekoot, C. Marcelletti & R.H. Anderson. Edinburgh: Churchill Livingstone.
Busquet, J., Davies, M.J., Anderson, R.H. & Fontan, F. (1984)

Surgical significance of the atrial branches of the coronary arteries. *International Journal of Cardiology*, **6**, 223–234.
Engel, H.J., Torres, C. & Page, H.L.Jr. (1975) Major variations in anatomical origin of the coronary arteries: angiographic observations in 4250 patients without associated congenital heart disease. *Catheterization and Cardiovascular Diagnosis*, **1**, 157–169.
Horiuchi, T., Abe, T., Tanaka, S. & Koyamada, K. (1971) Congenital coronary arteriovenous fistulas. *Annals of Thoracic Surgery*, **11**, 102–112.
Keeton, B.R., Keenan, D.J.M. & Monro, J.L. (1983) Anomalous

origin of both coronary arteries from the pulmonary trunk. *British Heart Journal*, **49**, 397–399.
Neufeld, H.N. & Schneeweiss, A. (1983) *Coronary Artery Disease in Infants and Children*, pp 73–75. Philadelphia: Lea & Febiger.
Rittenhouse, E.A., Doty, D.B. & Ehrenhaft, J.L. (1975) Congenital coronary artery-cardiac chamber fistula. Review of operative management. *Annals of Thoracic Surgery*, **20**, 468–485.

4 Surgical Anatomy of the Conduction System

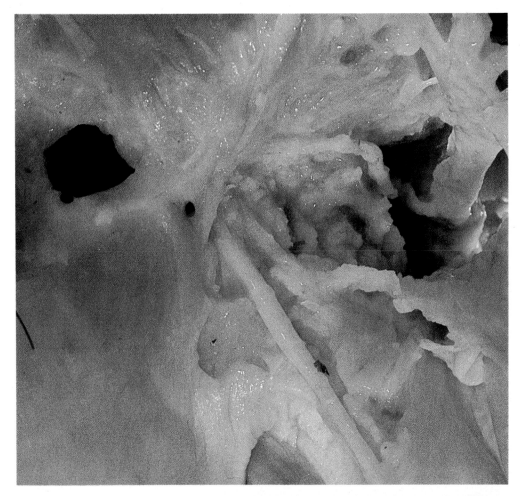

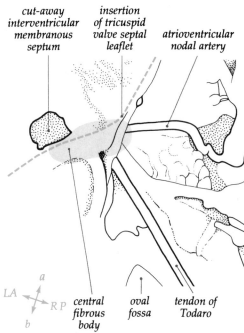

Fig. 4.1 *Right atrium dissected to show the tendon of Todaro. The interventricular component of the membranous septum has been excised.*

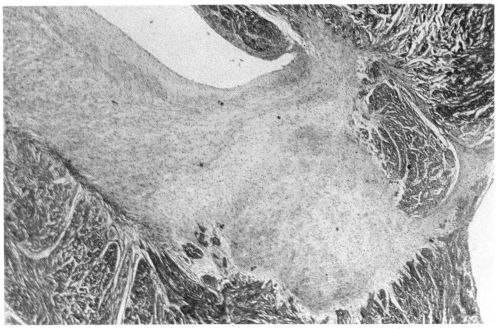

Fig. 4.2 *Histology of the penetrating atrioventricular bundle in surgical orientation. Trichrome stain.*

We have already discussed the disposition of the conduction system in the normal heart and described the importance of not only avoiding the cardiac nodes and ventricular bundle branches, but also the need to protect scrupulously the blood supply to these structures. In this chapter we will consider the surgical anatomy of these tissues in those patients who have intractable rhythm problems. Abnormal dispositions of conduction tissue secondary to congenital cardiac lesions will be discussed in the sections devoted to those lesions.

In patients with intractable tachycardia it may be necessary to ablate the atrioventricular bundle. Although this is sometimes accomplished accidentally when performing cardiac surgery, surprisingly it can be difficult to divide the bundle intentionally. The landmark to this structure is the apex of the triangle of Koch, the point at which the tendon of Todaro inserts into the central fibrous body (Fig. 4.1). At the apex of this triangle the axis of atrioventricular conduction tissue gathers itself together and enters the fibrous body (Fig. 4.2). It then

penetrates to the left through the fibrous body. In its course through the fibrous tissue it is crossed by the tricuspid valve septal leaflet as the latter structure itself divides the membranous septum into atrioventricular and interventricular components (Fig. 4.3). Having thus penetrated the septum, the branching bundle can usually be found sitting on the crest of the muscular septum immediately beneath the interventricular component of the membranous septum. When viewed from the left, the bundle is intimately related to the subaortic outflow

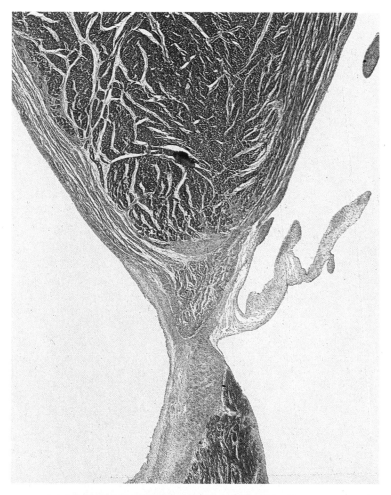

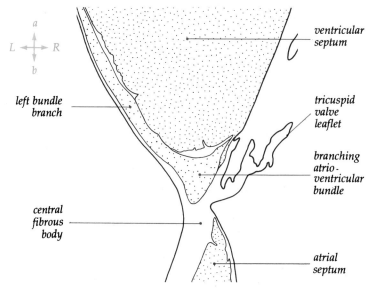

Fig. 4.3 *Histology of the tricuspid valve crossing the membranous septum in surgical orientation. The interventricular part of the membranous septum is occupied by the branching segment of the atrioventricular bundle. Trichrome stain.*

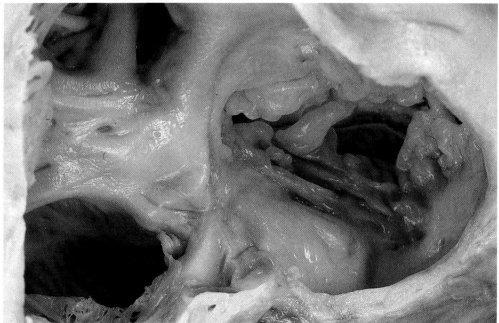

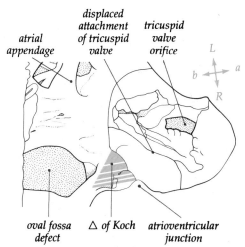

Fig. 4.4 *Right atrioventricular junction in surgical orientation in Ebstein's malformation. The triangle of Koch remains the guide to the site of the atrioventricular node. By courtesy of Mrs. Audrey Smith, Alder Hey Children's Hospital, Liverpool.*

tract; the non-coronary-right coronary commissure of the aortic valve is a good guide to its location. Sometimes the branching bundle lies below the septal crest, carried on the left ventricular aspect of the septum (*Massing & James, 1976*). From the left side the right bundle branch then burrows intramyocardially to reach the right side of the septum. These features taken together indicate that the apex of the triangle of Koch is the most appropriate marker for locating the bundle. The node itself within the triangle is some distance above the attachment of

the tricuspid valve septal leaflet and well anterior to the orifice of the coronary sinus. The apex of the triangle of Koch is of equal value as a landmark to the bundle in patients with Ebstein's anomaly (Fig. 4.4). This is noteworthy because Ebstein's anomaly is a quite frequent finding in patients with ventricular preexcitation, some of whom are very likely to require surgical division of the conduction tissue axis.

The surgical anatomy of ventricular preexcitation makes up the rest of this chapter. Preexcitation is the abnormal

cardiac rhythm in which all or part of the ventricular myocardium is excited earlier than would be expected had the impulse reached the ventricles by way of a normal atrioventricular conduction system (*Durrer, Schuilenburg & Wellens, 1970*). There are various anatomical pathways, proven and hypothetical, which could produce this phenomenon. In essence they are pathways which short-circuit part or all of the normal delay induced by the atrioventricular conduction tissues.

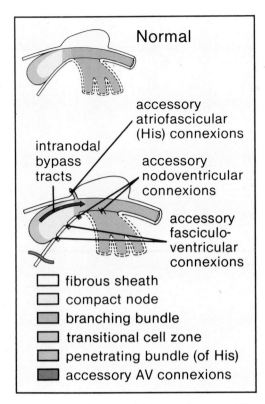

Normal

intranodal bypass tracts

accessory atriofascicular (His) connexions

accessory nodoventricular connexions

accessory fasciculo-ventricular connexions

☐ fibrous sheath
☐ compact node
▨ branching bundle
☐ transitional cell zone
▨ penetrating bundle (of His)
■ accessory AV connexions

Fig. 4.5 *Pathways which can circumvent the delay-producing area of the specialized conduction tissues and produce preexcitation.*

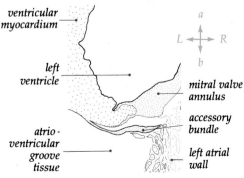

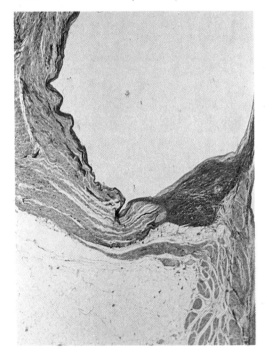

ventricular myocardium

left ventricle

atrio-ventricular groove tissue

a

L ←→ R

b

mitral valve annulus

accessory bundle

left atrial wall

Fig. 4.6 *Typical left-sided accessory atrioventricular connexion seen in surgical orientation. Elastic tissue stain. By courtesy of Prof. A.E. Becker.*

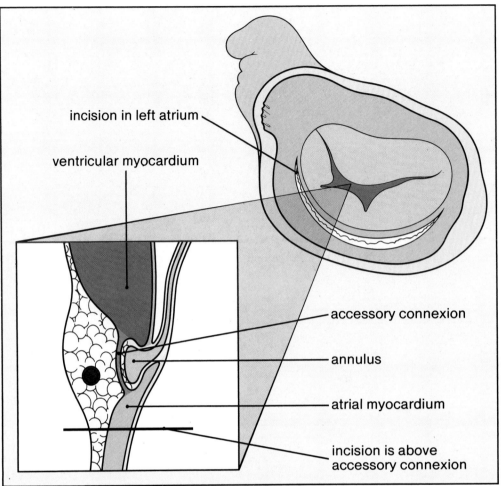

incision in left atrium

ventricular myocardium

accessory connexion

annulus

atrial myocardium

incision is above accessory connexion

Fig. 4.7 *Surgical view of incision advocated for ablation of preexcitation which does not sever the accessory connexion; (inset) section across the atrioventricular junction. Compare with Fig. 4.6.*

This delay is mostly effected within the atrioventricular node, but an increment is also imparted as the impulse traverses the ventricular conduction branches, these structures being insulated from the septal myocardium. The potential pathways which can circumvent this delay-producing area are shown diagrammatically in Fig. 4.5. Accessory pathways between the atrium and the atrioventricular bundle, between the conduction axis and the ventricular septum and the hypothetical pathways within the node are as yet not amenable to surgical division. However, the accessory atrioventricular pathways which produce the Wolff-Parkinson-White syndrome, probably the most common form of preexcitation, are very much amenable to surgical division (*Sealy, Gallagher & Pritchett, 1978; Sealy, 1983*). These pathways, often inappropriately called bundles of Kent (*Anderson & Becker, 1981*), connect the atrial and ventricular myocardial muscle masses outside the area of the specialized conduction tissues. They can be found anywhere around the atrioventricular junction and can be categorized conveniently as left-sided, right-sided and septal pathways. The anatomy of each group shows significant differences.

Left-sided pathways are found at any point around the mitral orifice, although

they are exceedingly rare in the area of aortic-mitral valve continuity. The pathways almost always run from atrial to ventricular muscle masses outside a well-formed fibrous annulus (Fig. 4.6). The atrial origin of the bundle is very close to the annulus and usually the bundle itself skirts very close to the annulus, often branching into several roots which then insert into the ventricular myocardium (*Becker et al., 1978*). The bundles are rarely thicker than one or two millimetres in diameter and are composed of ordinary myocardium. Frequently there may be more than one bundle in the same patient. The surgical significance of this anatomy is that incisions which divide the atrial myocardium above the mitral annulus are unlikely to divide the accessory muscle bundle itself. In order to ablate the accessory connexion it is usually necessary to dissect within the fat pad on the epicardial aspect of the annulus (Fig. 4.7).

Right-sided accessory pathways may also pass through the fat pad to connect the atrial and ventricular myocardial masses, but these are more frequently found some distance away from the tricuspid valve attachment. This attachment is rarely to a firm and well-formed annulus as on the mitral side (*Anderson & Becker, 1980*). This means that

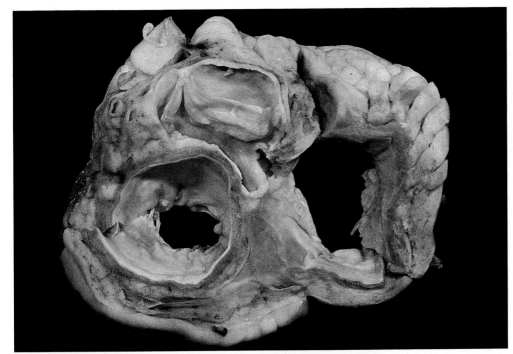

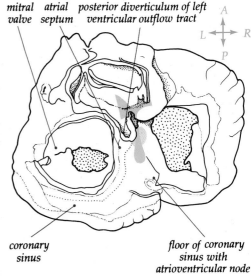

Fig. 4.8 *Short-axis view of the floor of the coronary sinus and its relationships. The site of the atrioventricular conduction axis is superimposed.*

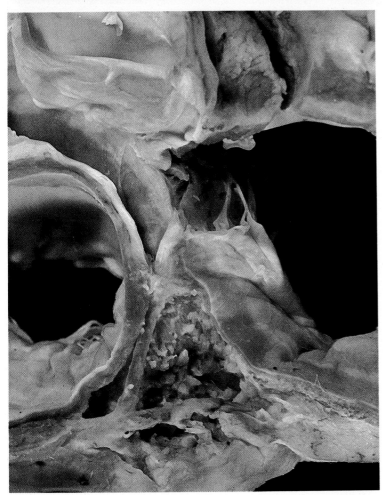

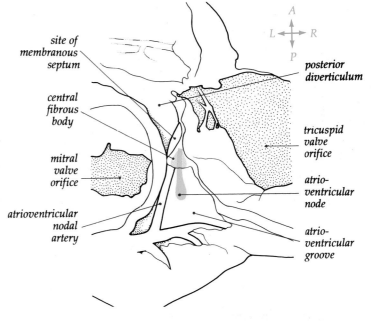

Fig. 4.9 *Coronary sinus floor showing the course of the atrioventricular nodal artery through an epicardial tissue plane. The site of the atrioventricular node is superimposed.*

because the annulus is less well-formed on the tricuspid side, the accessory connexions are also able to pass through the fibrous plane on its endocardial aspect. Right-sided connexions can be multiple and coexist with left-sided pathways. As already indicated they are frequently associated with Ebstein's malformation. They can be found at any point in the anterolateral aspect of the tricuspid orifice from the site of the membranous septum to the coronary

sinus. The same rules for their ablation apply as discussed for left-sided connexions except that it must be remembered that their pathways may pass along the endocardial as well as epicardial surface.

Septal connexions constitute the greatest surgical challenge (*Sealy & Gallagher, 1980*). When viewed from the right atrium, they can cross from the atrial to ventricular myocardium at any point in the septum between the coronary sinus and the membranous septum. They

present problems to the surgeon firstly because they may run deep within the septum as viewed from the right atrium, and secondly because the atrioventricular node and bundle are also found within this area. The anatomy of the area is best illustrated by a dissection of the floor of the coronary sinus (Fig. 4.8). This shows that a continuation of the atrioventricular groove extends beneath the sinus to reach the central fibrous body (Fig. 4.9). The artery to the atrioventricular node courses

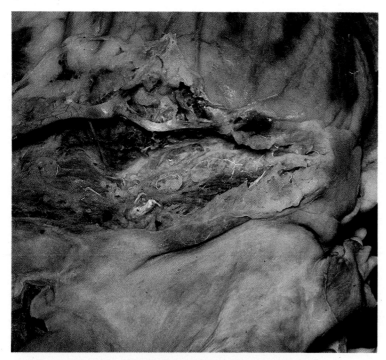

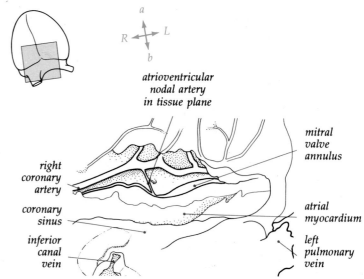

Fig. 4.10 *View of the posterior atrioventricular groove as would be seen if the apex of the heart were tilted upward, pivoting on the attachments of the inferior caval and pulmonary veins (inset). It shows the artery to the atrioventricular node.*

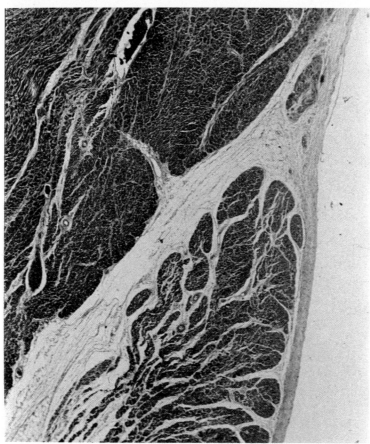

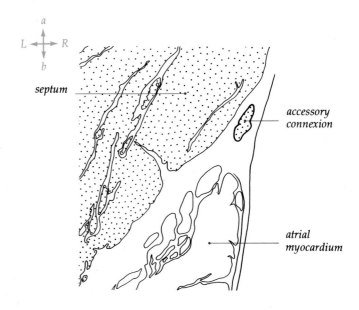

Fig. 4.11 *Histology of a septal accessory atrioventricular connexion crossing the adipose tissue plane at the distal extent of the right atrial myocardial insertion into the tricuspid valve leaflet. Trichrome stain. By courtesy of Prof. A.E. Becker.*

forwards within this tissue plane (Fig. 4.10) and the atrioventricular node itself occupies the anterior part (Fig. 4.9).

Accessory connexions may cross this plane at any point from the attachment of the mitral valve to the attachment of the tricuspid valve to the septum. Indeed, the only connexion we have identified within the septum (*Becker et al., 1978*) was located at the insertion of the tricuspid valve (Fig. 4.11). The tissue plane can be entered from the cavity of the right atrium, which is the approach advocated by Sealy and Gallagher (1980) for the division of these problematic connexions. However, the complex anatomy accounts for the relatively low success rate thus far achieved in accomplishing ablation without producing atrioventricular dissociation.

Anderson, R.H. & Becker, A.E. (1980) *Cardiac Anatomy. An Integrated Text and Colour Atlas*, pp 5.8–5.9. London, Edinburgh: Gower Medical Publishing–Churchill Livingstone.
Anderson, R.H. & Becker, A.E. (1981) Stanley Kent and accessory atrioventricular connexions. *Journal of Thoracic and Cardiovascular Surgery*, **81**, 649-658.
Becker, A.E., Anderson, R.H., Durrer, D. & Wellens, H.J.J. (1978) The anatomical substrates of Wolff-Parkinson-White syndrome: a clinico-pathologic correlation in seven patients. *Circulation*, **57**, 870-879.

Durrer, D., Schuilenburg, R.M. & Wellens, H.J.J. (1970) Pre-excitation revisited. *American Journal of Cardiology*, **25**, 690-698.
Massing, G.K. & James, T.N. (1976) Anatomical configuration of the His bundle and bundle branches in the human heart. *Circulation*, **53**, 609-621.
Sealy, W.C. (1983) Surgical treatment of two types of tachycardia caused by Kent bundles with only retrograde function. *Journal of Thoracic and Cardiovascular Surgery*, **85**, 746-751.

Sealy, W.C. & Gallagher, J.J. (1980) The surgical approach to the septal area of the heart based on experience with 45 patients with Kent bundles. *Journal of Thoracic and Cardiovascular Surgery*, **79**, 542-551.
Sealy, W.C., Gallagher, J.J. & Pritchett, E.L.C. (1978) The surgical anatomy of Kent bundles based on electro-physiological mapping and surgical exploration. *Journal of Thoracic and Cardiovascular Surgery*, **76**, 804-815.

5 Analytic Description of Congenitally Malformed Hearts

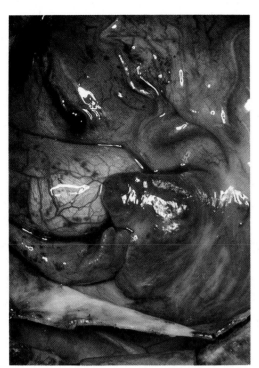
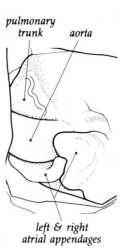

pulmonary
trunk   aorta

left & right
atrial appendages

Fig. 5.1 *Juxtaposition of the atrial appendages. Compare the broad triangular right appendage to the narrow constricted left appendage.*

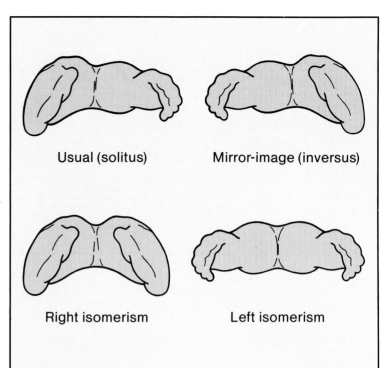

Usual (solitus)   Mirror-image (inversus)

Right isomerism   Left isomerism

Fig. 5.2 *The four possible atrial arrangements as determined by the morphology of their appendages.*

Previous systems for describing congenital cardiac malformations have frequently been based upon embryological concepts and theories. As useful as these systems have been, they have often had the effect of confusing the clinician rather than clarifying the basic anatomy of a given lesion. As far as the surgeon is concerned, the essence of a particular malformation lies not in its presumed morphogenesis but in the underlying anatomy. An effective system for describing this anatomy must be based upon the morphology as it is observed. At the same time, it must be capable of including all known congenital cardiac conditions. To be useful clinically the system must not only be broad and accurate but also clear and consistent. Therefore, the terminology used should be unambiguous, non-speculative and as simple as possible. Such a system is provided by the sequential segmental approach (*Anderson et al., 1984*). In this chapter we will describe this approach, emphasizing its surgical applications.

The basic philosophy of the system is to describe separately the connexions of the cardiac chambers, the morphology of the chambers and their interrelationships. This provides the basic framework within which all other associated malformations can be catalogued. For the surgeon it is the chamber connexions and morphology which are preeminent.

The first step in analyzing any congenitally malformed heart is to determine the arrangement of the atria. All atria are recognizable as being morphologically right or morphologically left in type, based on the anatomy of their atrial appendages. As described in Chapter 2, the morphologically right appendage has a broad triangular shape whereas the morphologically left appendage is much narrower and has several constrictions along its length (Fig. 5.1).

There are only four ways in which the atria can be arranged (Fig. 5.2). Almost always the atrium possessing the morphologically right appendage is right-sided and the morphologically left appendage is left-sided. This usual arrangement is generally called situs solitus. Rarely, the atria may be arranged in mirror-image fashion, situs inversus. More common that mirror-image atrial arrangement, but still rare, is where both appendages have the same morphology. This can occur in two forms, with morphologically right or morphologically left appendages on both sides. These bilaterally symmetrical arrangements (or isomeric types) have traditionally been named according to the abdominal viscera (*Van Mierop, Gessner & Schiebler, 1972; Stanger, Rudolph & Edwards, 1977*) as they usually exist with visceral heterotaxy. However, it is far more convenient to designate them in terms of their own intrinsic atrial morphology (*Macartney, Zuberbuhler & Anderson, 1980*), particularly since this can be readily determined by the surgeon at operation. Nonetheless, it is useful to know that right atrial isomerism is almost always found with asplenia and right bronchial isomerism while left atrial isomerism is found with polysplenia and left bronchial isomerism.

It should also be noted that atrial arrangement can be identified with a high degree of accuracy by studying the relationships of the abdominal great vessels with cross-sectional ultrasono-graphy (*Huhta, Smallhorn & Macartney, 1982*). Identification of atrial isomerism is of value in two additional ways. Firstly, it gives an indication of unusual dispositions of the sinus node. In right atrial isomerism the sinus node, being a morphologically right atrial structure, is duplicated. A node is found laterally in each of the terminal grooves (*Van Mierop & Wiglesworth, 1962*). In left atrial isomerism there are no terminal grooves and the sinus node is a poorly formed structure without a constant site. Usually it is found in the anterior inter-atrial groove close to the atrioventricular junction (*Dickinson et al., 1979*).

The second advantage of recognizing isomeric atria is that they are known to be frequently associated with other complex intracardiac lesions. Both forms tend to have bilateral superior caval veins, common atria and common atrio-ventricular valves. Right isomerism is almost invariably associated with total anomalous pulmonary venous connexion. It is also frequently seen with pulmonary stenosis or atresia and in hearts with a univentricular atrioventricular connexion. Left isomerism is associated with interruption of the inferior caval vein with azygos continuation in a majority of cases.

Having established the arrangement of the atria, it is then necessary to analyze the atrioventricular junction. For this one needs to know how the atria are (or are not) connected to the ventricles, the morphology of the valves which guard the atrioventricular junction and the morphology of the ventricles connected to the atria. We term the way in which the atria connect to the ventricles the type of atrioventricular connexion.

There are five distinct and discrete types

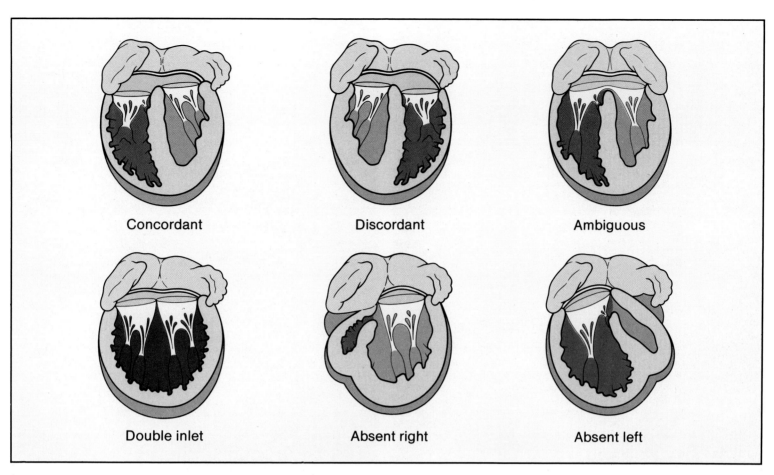

Concordant   Discordant   Ambiguous

Double inlet   Absent right   Absent left

Fig. 5.3 *The five possible types of atrioventricular connexion. The fifth variant (absent connexion) has two subtypes, absent right and absent left.*

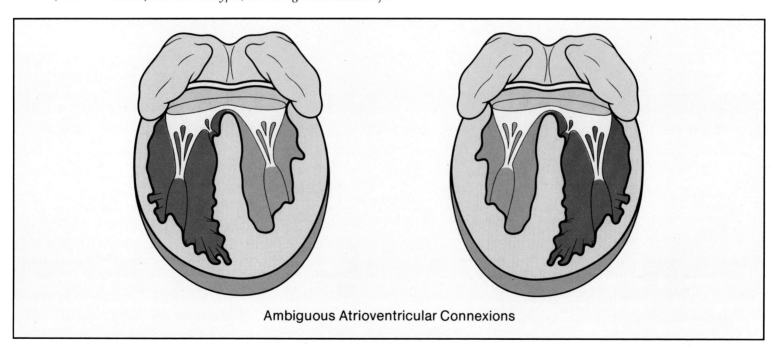

Ambiguous Atrioventricular Connexions

Fig. 5.4 *An ambiguous connexion can exist when the isomeric atrium is connected either to a morphologically right or a morphologically left ventricle.*

of connexion, the final one having two subtypes (Fig. 5.3). Most often, the morphologically right atrium is connected to the morphologically right ventricle and the morphologically left atrium to the morphologically left ventricle. This is termed atrioventricular concordance. When each atrium is connected in this way, there is rarely any difficulty in distinguishing the morphology of the ventricles, even when the chambers are unusually related (see below). In the second type of connexion, namely atrioventricular discordance, the morphologically right atrium connects with the morphologically left ventricle and the morphologically left atrium with the morphologically right ventricle.

Atrioventricular concordance and discordance can exist with either the usual or mirror-image arrangement of atria, but not with isomeric atria. When the atria are isomeric and each is connected to its own ventricle, of necessity half the connexion will be concordant but the other half will always be discordant (Fig. 5.4), irrespective of the ventricular topology (see below). This is a third type of connexion, namely an ambiguous atrioventricular connexion.

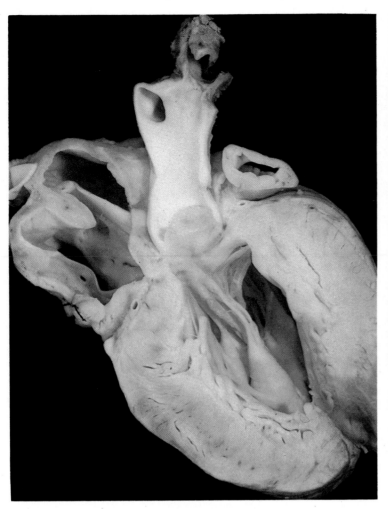

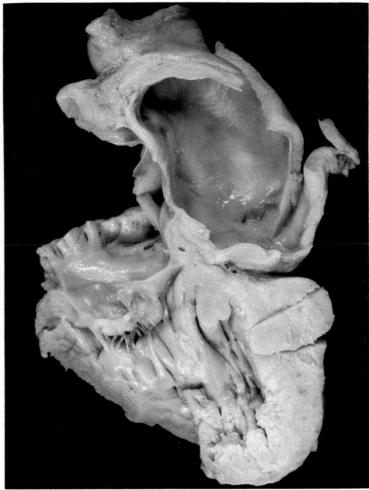

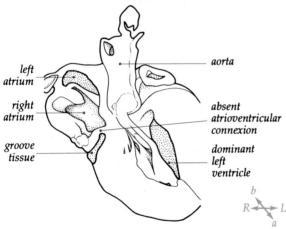

Fig. 5.5 *Long-axis view at right angles to the atrial septum ('four-chamber') of absent right atrioventricular connexion in a case of tricuspid atresia.*

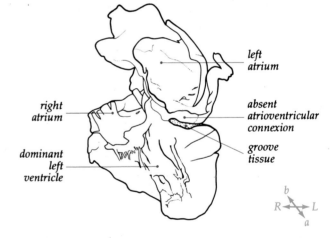

Fig. 5.6 *Long-axis 'four-chamber' view of absent left atrioventricular connexion. The right atrium is connected to a dominant left ventricle. By courtesy of Prof. G. Thiene, University of Padova.*

In the three connexions described thus far, each atrium is connected to its own ventricle. In the remaining two types of atrioventricular connexion the essential feature is that the atria connect to only a single ventricle. In one of these, both atria connect to the same ventricle, making a double inlet atrioventricular connexion. In the other, which has the two subtypes, one of the atria is connected to a ventricle but the other has no atrioventricular connexion at all. This is absence of one atrioventricular connexion. The two subtypes arise because the lack of connexion can be found in either the right (Fig. 5.5) or the left (Fig. 5.6) atrio-

ventricular junction.

Considerable controversy has been associated with hearts where the atria connect to only one ventricle, whether it be due to a double inlet or to absent connexion. Historically, such hearts have been classified as single ventricle, common ventricle or, more recently, as a univentricular heart. This is despite the fact that usually more than one chamber is present in the ventricular mass. By focusing on the fact that the atrioventricular connexion is to one ventricle only, a satisfactory solution is achieved for this dilemma in nomenclature, namely a univentricular atrioventricular

connexion. As one might anticipate, the ventricle connected to the atria can have one of three morphologies: right, left or indeterminate. Most frequently, the chamber connected to the atria will be a left ventricle as judged from its trabecular component. Almost always there will be a complementary right ventricle but without an atrioventricular connexion or inlet portion. Such rudimentary right ventricles are always found anterosuperior to the dominant left ventricle, irrespective of whether there is double inlet (Fig. 5.7), absent right (Fig. 5.8) or absent left (Fig. 5.9) atrioventricular connexion.

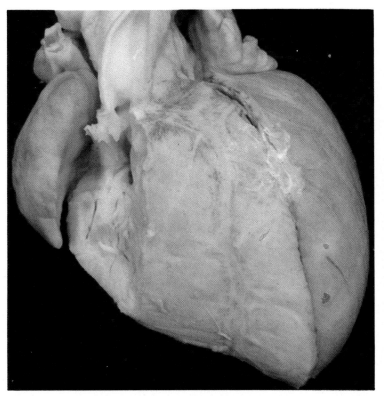

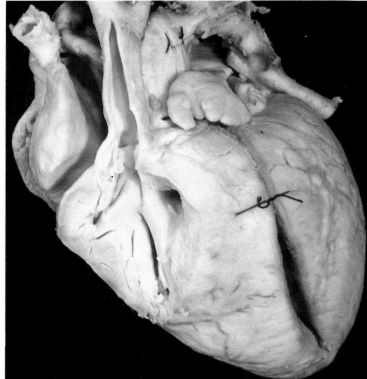

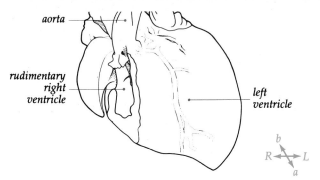

Fig. 5.7 *Anterior rudimentary right ventricle with double inlet to a dominant left ventricle. The rudimentary ventricle possesses only trabecular and outlet components.*

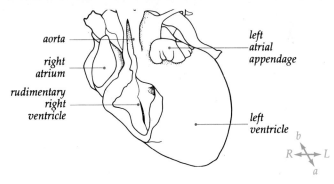

Fig. 5.8 *Anterior rudimentary right ventricle with absent right atrioventricular connexion with the left atrium connected to a dominant left ventricle. Compare with Fig. 5.7.*

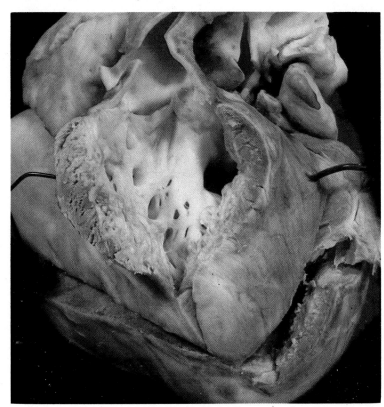

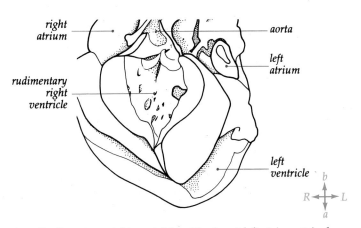

Fig. 5.9 *Rudimentary right ventricle with absent left atrioventricular connexion with the right atrium connected to a dominant left ventricle. Compare with Figs. 5.7 & 5.8.*

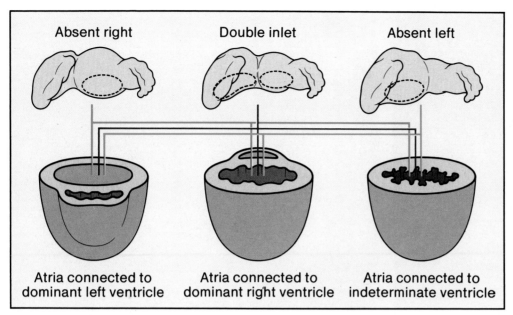

Fig. 5.10 *Combinations of connexions and ventricular morphology which produce variability in hearts with univentricular atrioventricular connexion.*

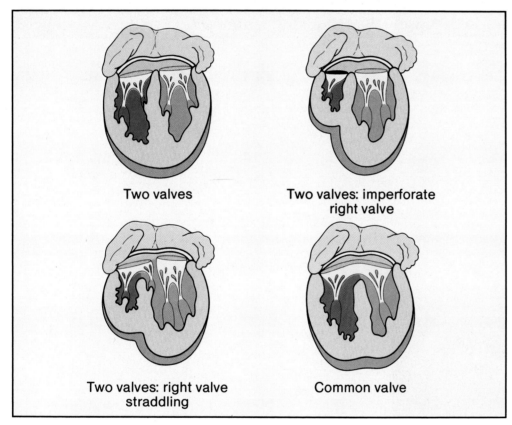

Fig. 5.11 *Modes of atrioventricular connexion.*

More rarely, the atria may be connected to a dominant right ventricle. This happens most frequently in the absence of the left atrioventricular connexion but can be found with double inlet or, rarely, with absent right atrioventricular connexion (Fig. 5.10). When only the right ventricle is connected to the atria, it is the left ventricle which almost always exists in rudimentary form, lacking an atrioventricular connexion and inlet portion. Invariably it will be found in a posteroinferior position, though it may be left-sided (usual) or right-sided (rare).

The third morphological configuration found with double inlet or, rarely, with absence of either atrioventricular connexion, is where the atria connect to a solitary ventricle of indeterminate morphology (Fig. 5.10). Rudimentary second ventricles are never found in this variant of univentricular atrioventricular connexion.

Atrioventricular valve morphology is independent of the type of connexion present and constitutes a separate feature which we call the mode of connexion (Fig. 5.11). With concordant, discordant, ambiguous or double inlet connexions there are always two atria connected to the ventricular mass. These two atrioventricular connexions can be guarded by two separate atrioventricular valves or by a common valve. When there are two valves, either can be imperforate. An imperforate valve must be distinguished from absence of an atrioventricular connexion since either can produce atrioventricular valve 'atresia'. With an imperforate valve, the connexion has formed but is blocked by a valve membrane (Fig. 5.12). When the connexion is absent, the floor of the involved atrium is completely separated from the ventricular mass by atrioventricular groove tissue (see Fig. 5.6).

Either of two valves or a common valve can also straddle a septum within the ventricular mass and this is another mode of connexion. We distinguish straddling of the tension apparatus of a valve from overriding of its annulus. Straddling is therefore present when the tension apparatus is attached to each side of a septum (Fig. 5.13). The degree of override, which usually coexists with straddling, determines the type of atrioventricular connexion present. For this purpose we assign the overriding valve to the ventricle connected to its greater part (the 'fifty percent law'; Fig. 5.14). The modes of connexion are much more limited when one atrioventricular connexion is absent. In this case the sole valve present can either be committed in its entirety to one ventricle or it can straddle.

From the above discussion it will be appreciated that the type of atrioventricular connexion is inextricably linked with ventricular morphology. Clearly, atrioventricular concordance or discordance cannot be defined until the ventricular morphology is known. On the other hand, although ambiguous, double inlet and absent connexions can all be identified without mention of ventricular morphology, it is always necessary to give more information concerning ventricular morphology. In the case of ambiguous connexion, the topology of the ventricular mass must be described, using the word 'topology' to specify the intrinsic arrangement of the morphologically right ventricle relative to the morphologically left ventricle. This is because the connexion is ambiguous when the isomeric atrium (of right or left morphology) is connected to either a morphologically right or a morphologically left ventricle (see Fig. 5.4). When a right-sided isomeric atrium is connected to a morphologically right ventricle, the ventricular mass is almost invariably as in hearts with atrioventricular concordance and usual atrial arrangement. In contrast, when a right-sided isomeric atrium is connected to a morphologically left ventricle, the ventricular mass is as usually found in the presence of atrioventricular discordance and usual atrial arrangement.

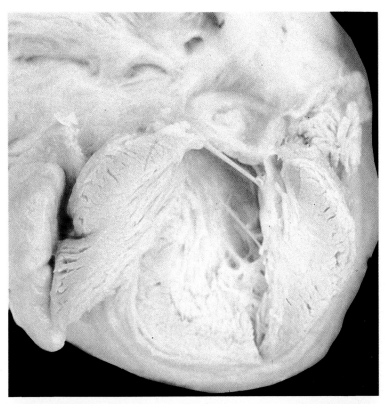

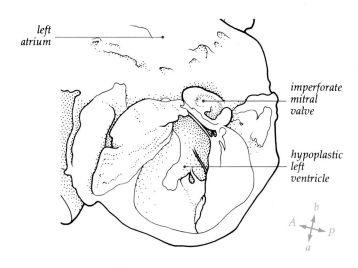

left atrium

imperforate mitral valve

hypoplastic left ventricle

A — P
b — a

Fig. 5.12 *Imperforate left atrioventricular valve in the setting of atrioventricular concordance. By courtesy of Dr. J.R. Zuberbuhler, Children's Hospital of Pittsburgh.*

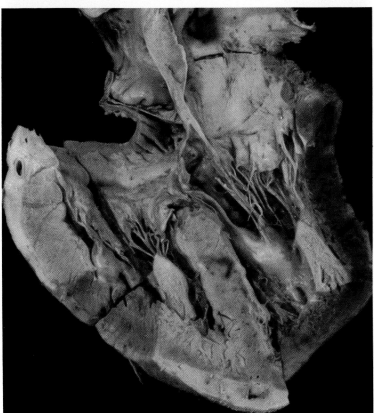

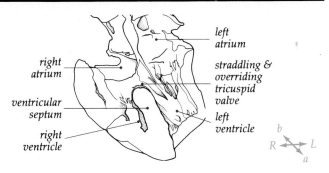

right atrium

left atrium

ventricular septum

straddling & overriding tricuspid valve

right ventricle

left ventricle

b — a
R — L

Fig. 5.13 *Long-axis 'four-chamber' view of a straddling and overriding right atrioventricular valve.*

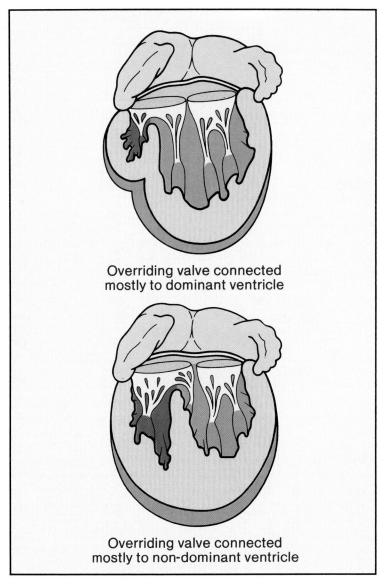

Overriding valve connected mostly to dominant ventricle

Overriding valve connected mostly to non-dominant ventricle

Fig. 5.14 *Extremes of the spectrum between univentricular and biventricular atrioventricular connexions found with overriding atrioventricular valves: (upper) double inlet connexion; (lower) biventricular connexion.*

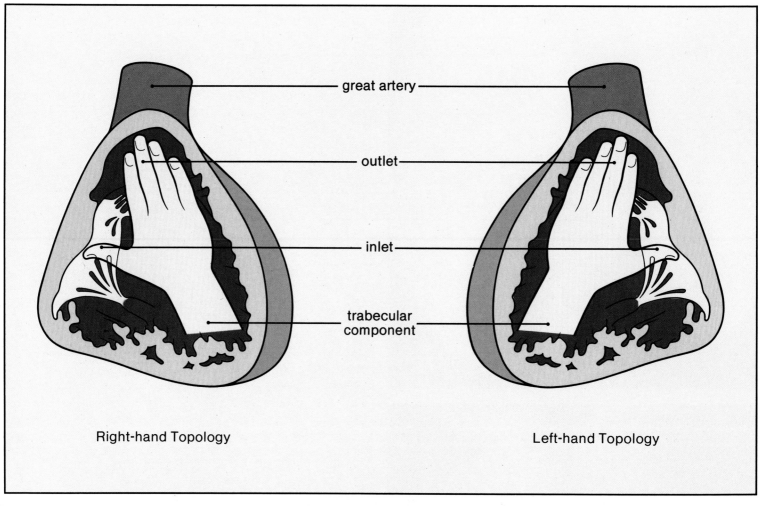

Fig. 5.15 *Patterns of ventricular topology can be compared to the palmar surfaces of the right and left hands when placed, figuratively speaking, on the morphologically right ventricular septal surface.*

These two basic patterns of topology can conveniently be described from the way in which a hand can be placed, figuratively speaking, palm downwards upon the morphologically right ventricular septal surface. When the ventricles are as typically found with the usual atrial arrangement and atrioventricular concordance, only the right hand can be placed so that the thumb is in the ventricular inlet and the fingers are in the outlet. When the usual atrial arrangement exists with atrioventricular discordance, only the left hand can be placed in this manner. These two patterns are respectively termed 'right-hand' and 'left-hand' patterns of ventricular topology (Fig. 5.15; *Van Praagh et al., 1980*). The significance of this feature in hearts with ambiguous connexion is that the ventricular topology determines the disposition of the atrioventricular conduction tissues (*Dickinson et al., 1979*; see below).

When the atria connect to only one ventricle its morphology must always be described because, as already stated, the dominant ventricle may be of left ventricular, right ventricular or indeterminate pattern. It is also necessary to determine if a coexistent rudimentary ventricle is present and to describe its

relationship to the dominant ventricle.

In general, ventricular relationships, as opposed to ventricular topology, should be described as a separate feature of the heart. However, where each atrium is connected to its own ventricle the relationships are almost always in harmony with both the connexion and topology present. Thus, when the atria are in their usual positions with atrioventricular concordance, the relationships described in the setting of the heart within the chest are almost always for the morphologically right ventricle to be right-sided, inferior and anterior to the morphologically left ventricle. In mirror-image atrial arrangement with atrioventricular concordance, the morphologically right ventricle is almost invariably left-sided, inferior and anterior to the morphologically left ventricle.

With atria in their usual arrangement and atrioventricular discordance, there is left-hand pattern ventricular topology and the usual relationship is for the morphologically right ventricle to be left-sided, inferior and anterior. When atrioventricular discordance accompanies mirror-image atria, there is right-hand topology and the ventricular relationships are similar to those in the normal heart. When the relationships are as

anticipated, it is unnecessary to describe them; but, very occasionally, the relationships of the ventricles are not as anticipated for the connexion present. These disharmonious relationships underscore the anomaly known as the 'criss-cross heart' (*Anderson, Shinebourne & Gerlis, 1974; Van Praagh et al., 1980*). With these hearts and also those with so-called 'superoinferior ventricles' (*Freedom, Culham & Rowe, 1978*), connexions and relationships must be described separately, using as much detail as necessary for unambiguous categorization. The essence of the 'criss-cross heart', therefore, is that the ventricular relationships are not as expected for the atrioventricular connexion present (Fig. 5.16).

In hearts with a univentricular atrioventricular connexion, the relationship of the rudimentary ventricle, if present, must be described. With a dominant left ventricle, the rudimentary ventricle is always anterosuperior but can be right- or left-sided. The sidedness of the ventricle does not affect the basic conduction tissue disposition in these hearts. With a dominant right ventricle, the rudimentary ventricle, if present, is always postero-inferior but again can be right- or left-sided. In this case the sidedness of the rudimentary ventricle does affect the

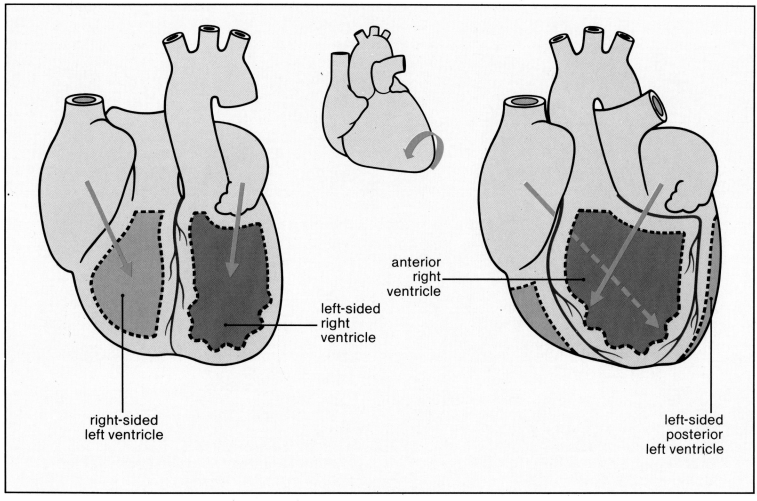

Fig. 5.16 *Rotational abnormality produces a 'criss-cross' heart in the setting of atrioventricular discordance: (left) anticipated relationships; (right) criss-cross arrangement produced by counter-clockwise rotation of the ventricular apex (inset).*

disposition of the conduction tissue (see below).

Thus, when considering the atrioventricular junction, there are four different features to take into account, namely the type and mode of connexion, the ventricular topology and the ventricular relationships. All are of importance to the surgeon because they influence the disposition of the atrioventricular conduction tissues. To appreciate the significance of these features it must be remembered that at one stage of development a complete ring of atrioventricular nodal tissue encircles the tricuspid orifice, sequestered on the atrial aspect by development of the fibrous annulus (Fig. 5.17). Usually the lateral parts of this ring neither function nor develop connexions with the ventricular conduction tissues. The part of the ring which persists is that within the atrial septum so that the definitive atrioventricular node is formed within the triangle of Koch, carried on the surface of the atrioventricular muscular septum. The ventricular components of the conduction tissue axis have different developmental origins. The penetrating and non-branching segments are formed in relation to the inlet part of the ventricular septum.

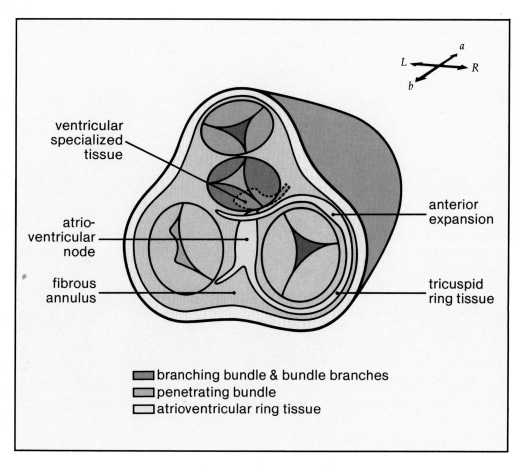

Fig. 5.17 *Ring of atrioventricular specialized conduction tissue in the fetal heart.*

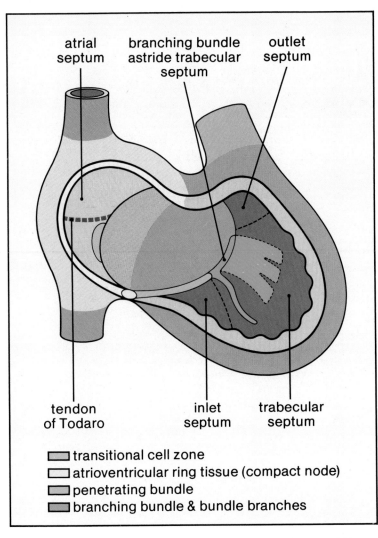

Fig. 5.18 *Segments of conduction tissue develop in relation to different septal structures.*

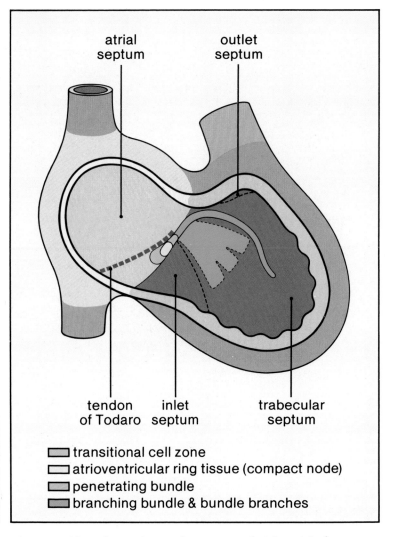

Fig. 5.19 *Normal septation produces a normal atrioventricular conduction tissue axis.*

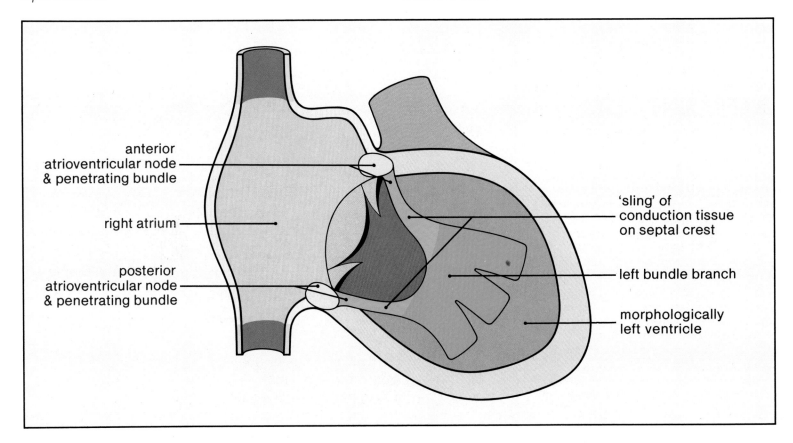

Fig. 5.20 *Right atrioventricular junction with atrioventricular discordance showing the site of the sling of conduction tissue which may be present.*

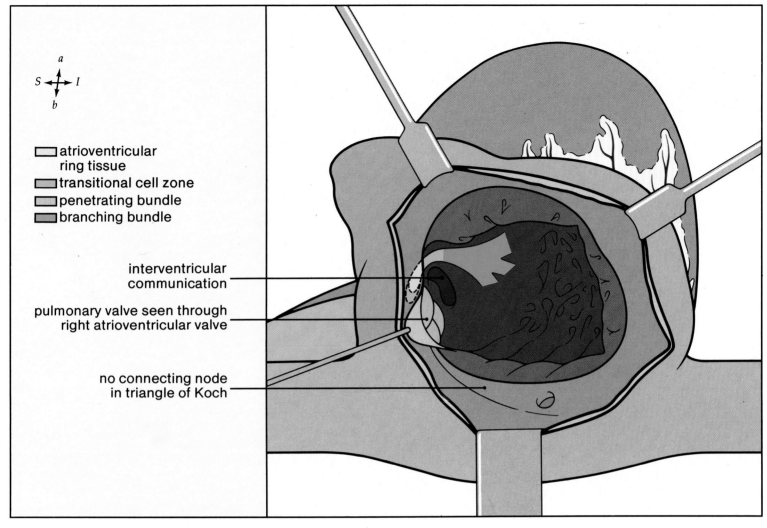

a
S ← → I
b

☐ atrioventricular
   ring tissue
▨ transitional cell zone
▨ penetrating bundle
▨ branching bundle

interventricular
communication

pulmonary valve seen through
right atrioventricular valve

no connecting node
in triangle of Koch

Fig. 5.21 *Operative view through the right atrioventricular valve showing the site of the anterior node and penetrating bundle in hearts with univentricular connexion to a left ventricle. The arrangement shown is found with left-sided rudimentary right ventricles (see Chapter 7).*

The branching bundle and the right and left bundle branches are formed astride the trabecular component of the septum (Fig. 5.18). Only with normal growth and alignment of these septal components is a normal conduction axis produced (Fig. 5.19). Normal disposition always occurs in the presence of atrioventricular concordance, except when the atrioventricular muscular septum is lacking (atrioventricular septal defects; see Chapter 6, iii) or when the tricuspid valve straddles and there is malalignment between the atrial and ventricular septa (see Chapter 6, iv).

Abnormal conduction tissue disposition is to be anticipated when abnormal connexions are found, particularly with a left-hand pattern of ventricular topology. For example, atrioventricular discordance is most often found with ventriculoarterial discordance, a combination which, with the usual atrial arrangement and almost invariably left-hand pattern of ventricular topology, produces gross malalignment of the atrial and ventricular septa and results in an anterior atrioventricular node and penetrating bundle. Even when there is good alignment between the atrial and ventricular septa with atrioventricular

discordance, there may be an abnormal conduction axis in posterior position or even a 'sling' of conduction tissue between the normal and anterior nodes (Fig. 5.20). A normal posterior arrangement is usual in atrioventricular discordance with mirror-image atria (*Wilkinson et al., 1978*) while slings can be found in atrioventricular discordance with double outlet right ventricle (*Monckeberg, 1913*).

In hearts with ambiguous atrioventricular connexion and right-hand pattern of ventricular topology there is a normal conduction tissue axis; but with a left-hand pattern our studies have always demonstrated a sling of conduction tissue (*Dickinson et al., 1979*). With univentricular atrioventricular connexions, septal orientation is the major determinant of the disposition of conduction tissue. To a lesser extent, the relationship of the rudimentary ventricle is influential. When the atria are connected only to a left ventricle, the inlet septum is always absent and the trabecular septum never extends to the crux. Therefore, there is always an anterior node in the atrioventricular orifice of the morphologically right atrium which gives rise to an anterior penetrating bundle (Fig.

5.21). This is found regardless of the relationship between the dominant left and rudimentary right ventricles. The only exception is when the morphologically right atrium has no connexion to the ventricular mass. Without an atrioventricular orifice there is nothing to separate the normal and anterior nodes. The result is the presence of a mass of nodal tissue in the floor of the blind-ending morphologically right atrium.

Where the atria connect only to a right ventricle, the ventricular septum does extend to the crux and the relationship of the rudimentary left ventricle is then significant. When the left ventricle is left-sided (right-hand ventricular topology), there is a normal connecting atrio-ventricular node. In the only case we have studied where the left ventricle was right-sided (left-hand topology), there was a sling of conduction tissue (*Essed et al., 1980*). Finally, in hearts with the atria connected to a solitary ventricle of indeterminate type, both inlet and trabecular septal components are lacking. Then, ordinarily, there is an anterior node, but the ventricular distribution of conduction pathways can be bizarre (*Becker, Wilkinson & Anderson, 1980*).

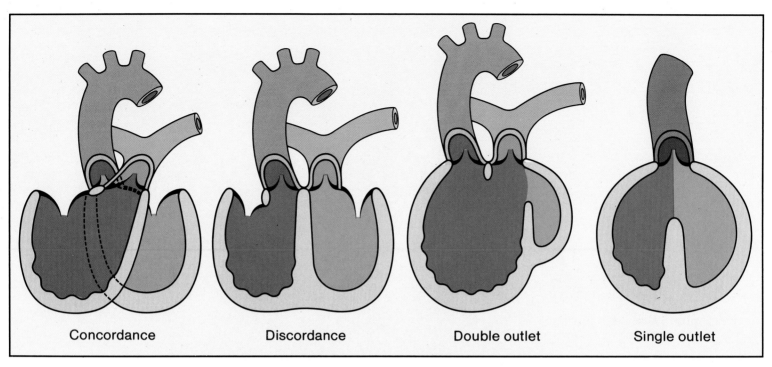

| Concordance | Discordance | Double outlet | Single outlet |

Fig. 5.22 *The four different types of ventriculoarterial connexion.*

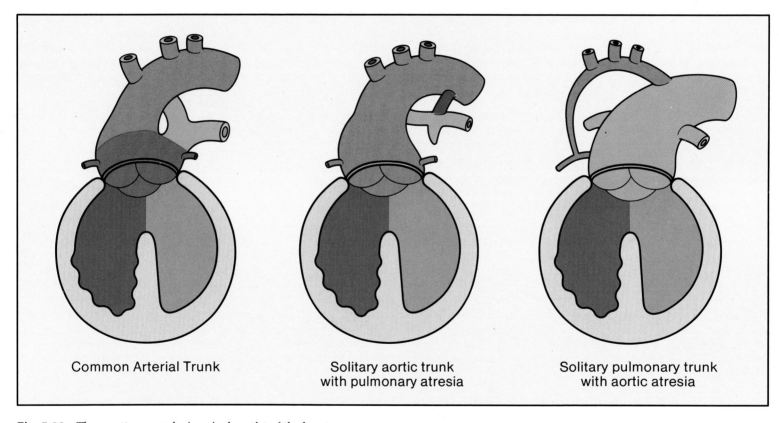

| Common Arterial Trunk | Solitary aortic trunk with pulmonary atresia | Solitary pulmonary trunk with aortic atresia |

Fig. 5.23 *Three patterns producing single outlet of the heart.*

Analysis of the ventriculoarterial junction proceeds as described for the atrioventricular junction, with type and mode of connexion, morphology and relationships being different facets requiring separate description in mutually exclusive terms.

There are four discrete types of ventriculoarterial connexion, namely concordance, discordance, double outlet and single outlet (Fig. 5.22). Ventriculoarterial concordance exists when the aorta is connected to a morphologically left ventricle and the pulmonary trunk to a morphologically right ventricle. Ventriculoarterial discordance describes connexion of the aorta to a morphologically right ventricle and the pulmonary trunk to a morphologically left ventricle. A double outlet connexion exists when both great arteries are connected to the same ventricle, which may be of right, left or indeterminate morphology. Finally, single outlet is the arrangement in which only one arterial trunk is connected to the heart (Fig. 5.23). This may be a common trunk, supplying directly the systemic, pulmonary and coronary arteries or it may be a single aortic or pulmonary trunk when the complementary arterial trunk is atretic and its connexion to a known ventricle cannot be established (Fig. 5.24).

The modes of ventriculoarterial connexion are limited because an arterial valve has an annulus but no tension apparatus. A common valve can only exist with a common trunk and is an integral part of the connexion. The different modes of ventriculoarterial connexion therefore involve one of two arterial valves. Usually both valves are perforate, but either or both may override

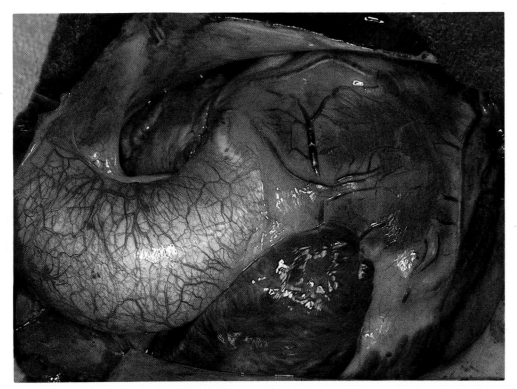

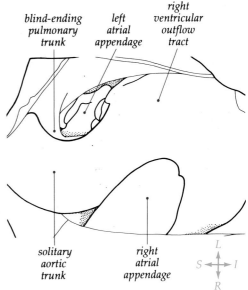

blind-ending
pulmonary
trunk

left
atrial
appendage

right
ventricular
outflow
tract

solitary
aortic
trunk

right
atrial
appendage

L
S ← → *I*
R

Fig. 5.24 *Operative view of a solitary aortic trunk with pulmonary atresia. Since the ventricular origin of the atretic trunk cannot be determined, it is more accurate to call this a single outlet ventriculoarterial connexion.*

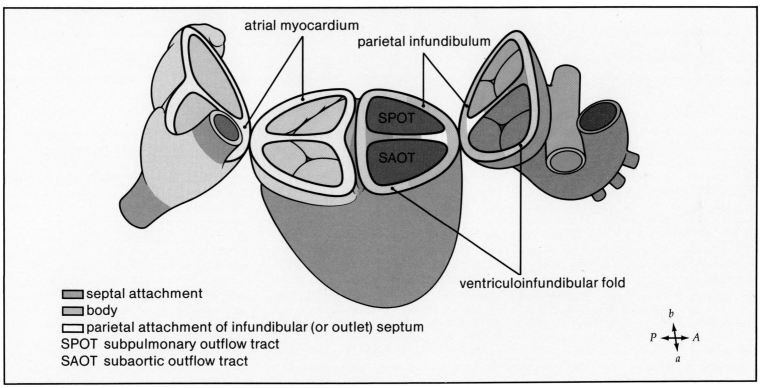

atrial myocardium

parietal infundibulum

SPOT

SAOT

ventriculoinfundibular fold

▭ septal attachment
▭ body
▭ parietal attachment of infundibular (or outlet) septum
SPOT subpulmonary outflow tract
SAOT subaortic outflow tract

b
P ← → *A*
a

Fig. 5.25 *Idealized double outlet right ventricle with right-sided aorta showing what would be seen if the atria and great arteries were hinged respectively on the posterior and anterior aspects of the ventricular mass. A complete cone of musculature supports the aortic and pulmonary valves with parietal, septal and inner curve (ventriculoinfundibular fold) segments.*

the ventricular septum. With overriding, we again apply the 'fifty percent law' and assign the valve to the ventricle connected to its greater part, thus avoiding the need for intermediate categories.

The other mode of connexion is when one of the arterial valves is imperforate. As with the atrioventricular junction, an imperforate arterial valve (mode of connexion) must be distinguished from absence of a ventriculoarterial connexion (type of connexion) since both can

produce arterial valve 'atresia'.

Description of morphology at the ventriculoarterial junction involves the anatomy of the ventricular outflow tracts, in other words, 'infundibular' morphology. Although the outlet regions are integral parts of the ventricular mass, it is traditional to consider them with the great arteries. Indeed, some authorities use ventricular outlet morphology as the criterion of a ventriculoarterial connexion, but we do not recommend this. The two

outflow tracts together make a complete cone of musculature with a parietal component, a septal component and a component adjacent to the atrioventricular junction (Fig. 5.25). The parietal component is the anterior free wall of whichever ventricle supports the infundibulum. The septal component is the infundibular septum which has a body with septal and parietal insertions. The component adjacent to the atrioventricular junction always separates an arterial valve

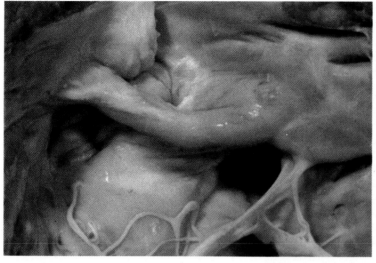

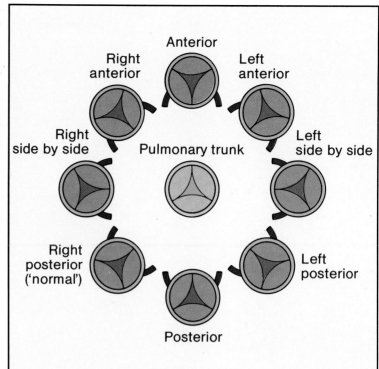

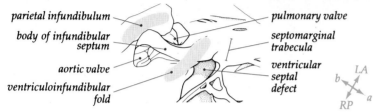

parietal infundibulum

body of infundibular septum

aortic valve

ventriculoinfundibular fold

pulmonary valve

septomarginal trabecula

ventricular septal defect

Fig. 5.26 *Outlet morphology seen from the right ventricular apex of double outlet right ventricle with bilateral infundibulum showing the different muscular structures.*

Fig. 5.27 *Combinations of anterior-posterior and right-left coordinates used to describe the interrelationships of the aortic and pulmonary valves.*

from an atrioventricular valve, and we term this structure the ventriculo-infundibular fold (Fig. 5.26).

None of the infundibular structures ever contain or overlie conduction tissue so it is vital to distinguish them from another structure, namely the septomarginal trabecula or 'septal band', which is part of the ventricular septum and reinforces its right ventricular aspect. It has a body that continues apically as the moderator band, and two 'limbs'. The anterior limb extends to the pulmonary valve overlying the outlet septum, and the posterior limb runs backwards beneath the interventricular membranous septum to connect with the inlet septum (see Fig. 2.30). This posterior limb usually overlies the branching part of the atrioventricular bundle while the right bundle branch passes down to the apex within the body of the trabecula.

Returning to the structure of the outflow tracts, both of these are potentially complete muscular structures, but usually only the outflow tract of the right ventricle is a complete muscular cone. This is because, within the left ventricle, part of the ventriculoinfundibular fold is usually attenuated to produce atrioventricular-arterial valve fibrous continuity. In the

normal heart, therefore, there is a muscular subpulmonary infundibulum in the right ventricle and fibrous aortic-atrioventricular valve continuity in the left ventricle.

In congenitally malformed hearts, three other patterns may be found: a muscular subaortic infundibulum with pulmonary-atrioventricular continuity, a bilaterally muscular infundibulum and a bilaterally deficient infundibulum. In the presence of a truncus, there may be a complete muscular subtruncal infundibulum, but more often there is a truncal-atrioventricular valve continuity.

The final feature of consideration at the ventriculoarterial junction is the relationship of the arterial valves and great arteries. Valve relationships are independent of both ventriculoarterial connexions and infundibular morphology. Of the many methods of description, our preference is to describe the aortic valve relative to the pulmonary valve as viewed from below in right-left, anterior-posterior and, when necessary, superior-inferior coordinates. This can be done as precisely as required but, in our experience, eight coordinates combining lateral and anterior-posterior positions suffice (Fig.

5.27). When describing the relationship of the arterial trunks it is sufficient to account for trunks which spiral round each other as they ascend and to distinguish them from parallel trunks.

The system discussed in this chapter establishes the cardiac template, but it is well known that the heart itself occupies a variable position, particularly when there are complex intracardiac malformations. To describe cardiac position it is necessary to account separately for the site of the heart within the thorax and the orientation of its apex. Our preference is to describe the heart as being in the left or right side of the chest or in the midline. Apex orientation is described as being to the left, to the middle or to the right.

Finally, having described the cardiac template and position, it is necessary to catalogue all intracardiac malformations. In most cases these lesions constitute the 'meat' of a given case; but any lesion, however simple, cannot be presumed to be the only lesion until the rest of the heart has been established as normal. It is on these associated lesions that we will henceforth concentrate, taking particular note, as before, of the features of surgical significance.

Anderson, R.H., Becker, A.E., Freedom, R.M., Macartney, F.J., Quero-Jimenez, M., Shinebourne, E.A., Wilkinson, J.L. & Tynan, M.J. (1984) Sequential segmental analysis of congenital heart disease. *Pediatric Cardiology* (in press).

Anderson, R.H., Shinebourne, E.A. & Gerlis, L.M. (1974) Criss-cross atrioventricular relationships producing paradoxical atrioventricular concordance or discordance. Their significance to nomenclature of congenital heart disease. *Circulation*, **50**, 176–180.

Becker, A.E., Wilkinson, J.L. & Anderson, R.H. (1980) Atrioventricular conduction tissues: a guide in understanding the morphogenesis of the univentricular heart. In *Etiology and Morphogenesis of Congenital Heart Disease*, pp 489–514. Edited by R. Van Praagh & A. Takao. Mount Kisco, New York: Futura Publishing Company.

Dickinson, D.F., Wilkinson, J.L., Anderson, K.R., Smith, A., Ho, S.Y. & Anderson, R.H. (1979) The cardiac conduction system in situs ambiguus. *Circulation*, **59**, 879–885.

Essed, C.E., Ho, S.Y., Hunter, S. & Anderson, R.H. (1980) Atrioventricular conduction system in univentricular heart of right ventricular type with right-sided rudimentary chamber. *Thorax*, **35**, 123–127.

Freedom, R.M., Culham, G. & Rowe, R.D. (1978) The criss-cross heart and superoinferior ventricular heart: an angiocardiographic study. *American Journal of Cardiology*, **42**, 620–628.

Huhta, J.C., Smallhorn, J.F. & Macartney, F.J. (1982) Two-dimensional echocardiographic diagnosis of situs. *British Heart Journal*, **48**, 97–108.

Macartney, F.J., Zuberbuhler, J.R. & Anderson, R.H. (1980) Morphological considerations pertaining to recognition of atrial isomerism. Consequences for sequential chamber localisation. *British Heart Journal*, **44**, 657–667.

Monckeberg, J.G. (1913) Zur Entwicklungsgeschichte des Atrioventrikularsystems. *Verhandlung der deutschen Pathologischen Gesellschaft*, **16**, 228–249.

Stanger, P., Rudolph, A.M. & Edwards, J.E. (1977) Cardiac malpositions: an overview based on study of sixty-five necropsy specimens. *Circulation*, **56**, 159–172.

Van Mierop, L.H.S., Gessner, I.H. & Schiebler, G.L. (1972) Asplenia and polysplenia syndromes. In *Birth Defects: Original Article Series*, **8**:5, pp 36–44. Baltimore: Williams & Wilkins.

Van Praagh, S., LaCorte, M., Fellows, K.E., Bossina, K., Busch, H.J., Keck, E.W., Weinberg, P.M. & Van Praagh, R. (1980) Superoinferior ventricles: anatomic and angiographic findings in ten post-mortem cases. In *Etiology and Morphogenesis of Congenital Heart Disease*, pp 317–378. Edited by R. Van Praagh & A. Takao. Mount Kisco, New York: Futura Publishing Company.

Wilkinson, J.L., Smith, A., Lincoln, C. & Anderson, R.H. (1978) The conducting tissues in congenitally corrected transposition with situs inversus. *British Heart Journal*, **40**, 41–48.

6 Lesions in Normally Connected Hearts

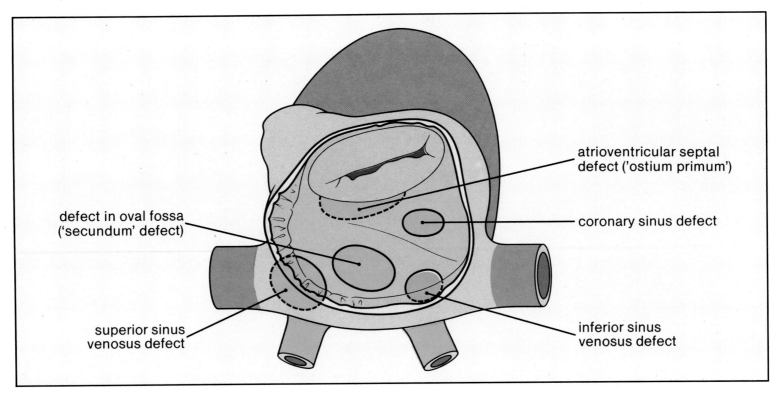

Fig. 6.1 *Different sites of interatrial communications. Only the defect within the oval fossa is a true atrial septal defect.*

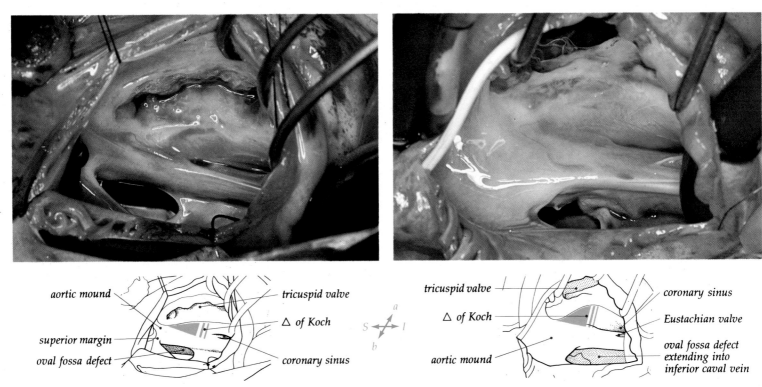

Fig. 6.2 *Operative view of typical defect at the site of the oval fossa ('secundum' defect).*

Fig. 6.3 *Operative view of oval fossa defect extending towards the mouth of the inferior caval vein.*

i. Atrial septal defects

There are several lesions which permit interatrial shunting (Fig. 6.1). Although collectively termed 'atrial septal defects', they are not all within the confines of the normal atrial septum (see Fig. 2.12). In fact, only the so-called secundum defect is a true atrial septal defect. The ostium primum defect is due to a deficiency of the atrioventricular septum and will be considered in the next section. The sinus venosus defects, most frequently associated

with partial anomalous pulmonary venous drainage, are found at the mouths of the caval veins. Finally, there is the defect of the orifice of the coronary sinus where the sinus itself is unroofed.

The secundum defect is by far the most common. It is at the site of the oval fossa and is usually due to deficiency of perforation of the floor (the flap-valve of the foramen). Although the haemodynamics dictate surgical closure, the hole of a defective fossa is unlikely to be small

enough to permit direct suture. If attempted, the results may so distort atrial anatomy as to result in dehiscence. Since the edge of the fossa is almost always intact and has no surgically vulnerable structures, a patch can be readily secured to its margins. The only potential dangers (Fig. 6.2) are to the sinus node artery, which sometimes courses intramyocardially through the superior margin, and to the aorta, which underlies the anterior margin (the aortic mound). In

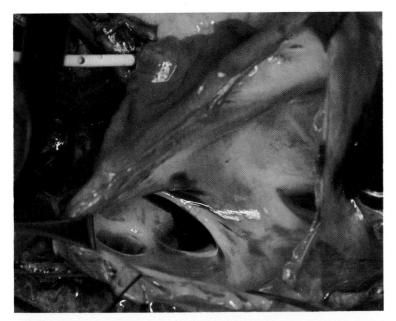

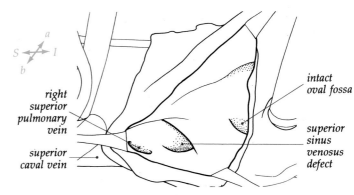

Fig. 6.4 *Superior cavoatrial junction opened surgically to show a sinus venosus defect.*

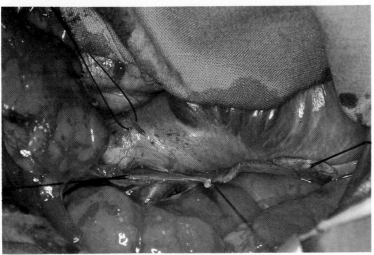

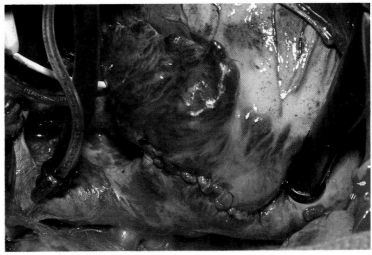

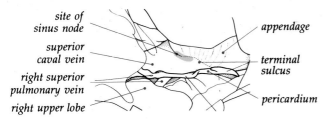

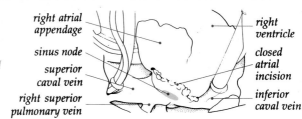

Fig. 6.5 *Operative view of same heart as in Fig. 6.4 showing the anomalous course of the right superior pulmonary vein and the site of the sinus node.*

Fig. 6.6 *Incision used to gain access to the right atrium for repair of the sinus venosus defect is well away from the site of the sinus node.*

some cases the posteroinferior edge of the fossa is deficient, extending the defect into the mouth of the inferior caval vein (Fig. 6.3). It is possible to mistake a well formed Eustachian valve for the postero-inferior margin of the defect. Because a patch attached to this valve would connect the inferior caval vein to the left atrium, it is always prudent to ensure continuity of the inferior caval vein and right atrium following placement of the patch.

Sinus venosus defects are rarer than secundum defects and present greater problems in repair. The inferior sinus venosus defect is extremely rare. It opens into the mouth of the inferior caval vein posterior to the confines of the oval fossa, which is usually intact. The right inferior pulmonary vein is usually in close

proximity to the interatrial defect. The problems of closure relate to ensuring that the venous drainage is routed to the appropriate atrium.

The sinus venosus defect at the mouth of the superior caval vein is much more frequently seen (Fig. 6.4). It, too, is outside the confines of the oval fossa and may be intimately related to the orifice of the right superior pulmonary vein. Indeed, the vein frequently drains directly into the superior caval vein (Fig. 6.5) and often through more than one orifice. The major difficulty here is constructing a repair which reroutes the venous return and closes the interatrial defect without obstructing superior caval venous return or damaging the sinus node. As described in Chapter 2, the sinus node is related to

the anterolateral quadrant of the cavoatrial junction and lies immediately sub-epicardially within the terminal sulcus (Fig. 6.5). The sinus node should not be at risk with simple closure (Fig. 6.6). The problem arises with the necessity either to suture in the area of the node when rerouting the pulmonary venous return or to enlarge the orifice of the caval vein. The former risk can be minimized with judicious placement of the sutures; the latter problem is much greater. Because the artery to the sinus node may pass either in front of or behind the caval vein, the entire cavoatrial junction is a potentially dangerous area. Determining the course of the nodal artery beforehand would facilitate the design of an operation least likely to damage the node or its artery.

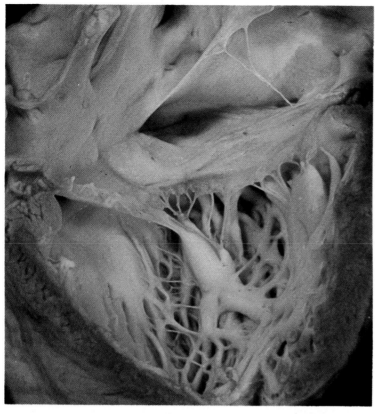

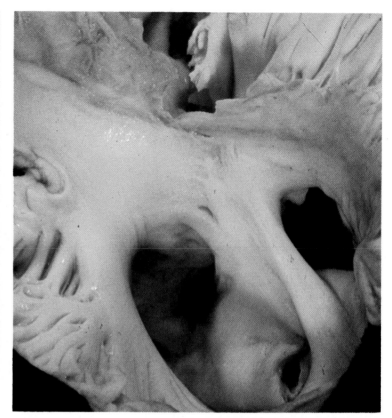

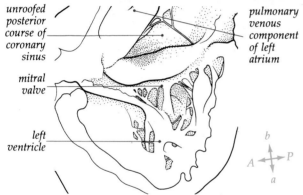

Fig. 6.7 *Left superior caval vein draining directly to the left atrium with unroofing of its posterior course. The parietal part of the left atrioventricular junction has been opened.*

Fig. 6.8 *Orifice of the unroofed coronary sinus, which now permits interatrial communication, in surgical orientation.*

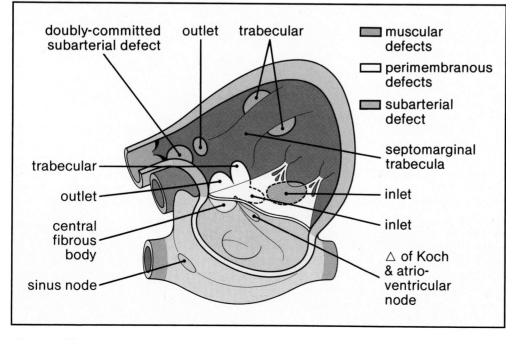

Fig. 6.9 *The various sites of ventricular septal defects as would be seen by the surgeon.*

The final defect which permits interatrial shunting is part of a constellation of lesions and is probably best termed 'unroofed coronary sinus' (*Quaegebeur et al., 1979*). In this combination, a persistent left superior caval vein drains directly to the left atrial roof between the appendage and the left pulmonary veins (Fig. 6.7) and there is a large hole at the site of the coronary sinus (Fig. 6.8). Usually, there is morphological evidence of the course the vein should have taken between the atrial roof and the left side of the orifice of the coronary sinus. Surgical treatment depends upon the connexions of this persistent left caval vein. If it is in free communication with the right superior caval vein, the left-sided channel can simply be ligated and the orifice of the coronary sinus closed. If the left-sided channel has no anastomoses with the right side, it may be better to construct a channel in the posterior wall of the left atrium.

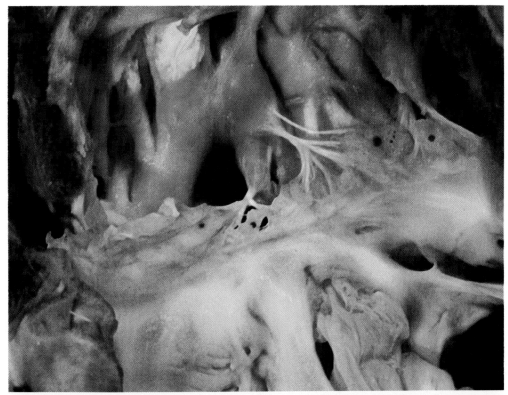

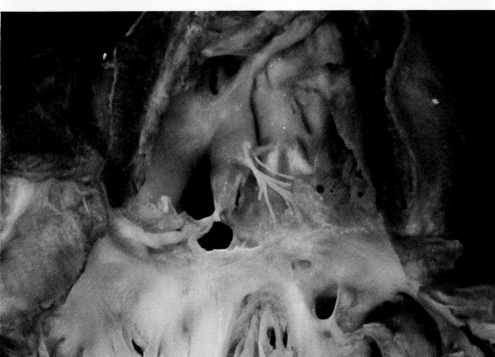

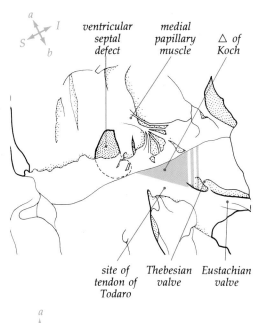

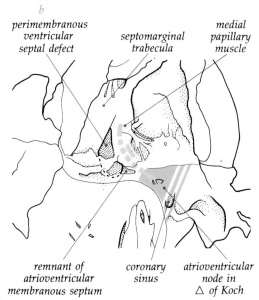

Fig. 6.10 *Basic features of perimembranous defect and typical course of atrioventricular conduction tissue axis seen before (upper) and after (lower) removal of the septal leaflet of the tricuspid valve, in surgical orientation.*

ii. Ventricular septal defects

When faced with a clinically significant ventricular septal defect, the primary concern of the surgeon is whether he can effect a safe and secure closure. The important anatomical considerations relate to the location of the defect within the ventricular septum, as this determines its proximity to the atrioventricular conduction axis and atrioventricular and arterial valves. The categorization of ventricular septal defects proposed by Soto et al. (1980) is invaluable in that it focuses the attention of the surgeon on these pertinent features. In short, Soto and his colleagues suggested that defects could be considered as perimembranous, muscular or doubly-committed subarterial

and that the first two groups could be further described as being located primarily within the inlet, trabecular or outlet parts of the septum (Fig. 6.9).

The essence of a perimembranous defect is that a part of the central fibrous body, made up of mitral-aortic-tricuspid valve continuity, forms part of its rim. The defects are termed 'perimembranous' rather than 'membranous' because the atrioventricular component of the membranous septum is always present in the rim of the defect as part of the central fibrous body, and because the inter-ventricular component is frequently found as a fold of fibrous tissue in the rim.

The defect itself results from a deficiency of muscular tissue around the

membranous components (*Becu et al., 1956*). Indeed, defects requiring surgical closure will always be considerably larger than the area occupied by the interventricular membranous septum of the normal heart. This morphology has important consequences for conduction tissue disposition. As described in Chapter 4, the conduction axis penetrates through the atrioventricular membranous septum to reach the crest of the muscular septum immediately beneath the inter-ventricular membranous septum (see Fig. 4.3). In perimembranous defects, therefore, the axis penetrates through the area of aortic-tricuspid valve continuity (Fig. 6.10).

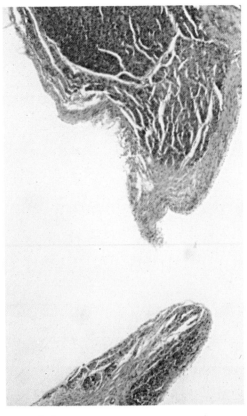

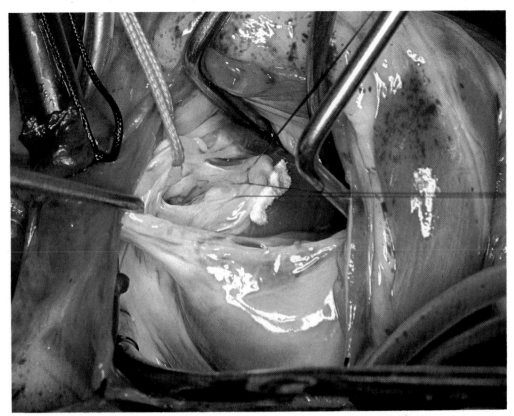

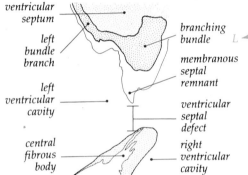

ventricular septum

left bundle branch

left ventricular cavity

central fibrous body

branching bundle — L ← a → R

membranous septal remnant — b

ventricular septal defect

right ventricular cavity

Fig. 6.11 *Histological section showing the non-branching atrioventricular bundle encased in a remnant of the membranous septum in a perimembranous ventricular septal defect, in surgical orientation. Trichrome stain.*

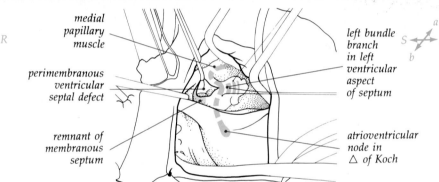

medial papillary muscle

perimembranous ventricular septal defect

remnant of membranous septum

left bundle branch in left ventricular aspect of septum — S ← a → I, b

atrioventricular node in △ of Koch

Fig. 6.12 *Operative view through tricuspid valve showing relationship of the conduction tissue axis to a perimembranous ventricular septal defect. The remnant of interventricular membranous septum lies directly on top of the non-branching bundle.*

When an interventricular membranous remnant is present, it lies immediately on top of the conduction bundle (Fig. 6.11). If such a remnant is seen at operation (Fig. 6.12), it should be appreciated that it is not a safe anchorage for deeply placed sutures.

These landmarks, together with the apex of the triangle of Koch as the atrial guide to the site of penetration, are useful for all types of perimembranous defects (*Milo et al., 1980*). However, the proximity to the aortic and atrioventricular valves varies, depending upon the precise area of deficiency in the muscular septum. In all cases, it is likely that the inlet, trabecular and outlet components are all deficient in part and, usually, it can be determined which part is most affected.

When a perimembranous defect extends mostly into the inlet septum (Fig. 6.13), its atrial margin (as viewed through the tricuspid valve) is an extensive area of

mitral-tricuspid valve continuity. The apex of the triangle of Koch is usually deviated towards the coronary sinus (the surgeon's right hand) and the bundle penetrates through this corner of the defect. Usually, the non-branching and branching bundles are carried on the left ventricular aspect as they descend the right-hand margin of the defect. The right bundle branch then courses intramyocardially, surfacing beneath the medial papillary muscle, which is usually at the left-hand margin. The non-coronary leaflet of the aortic valve is more to the left and usually distant from the rim of the defect.

When a perimembranous defect extends mostly into the trabecular septum, its orientation is more towards the ventricular apex. The triangle of Koch is not deviated as far towards the coronary sinus but the right-hand rim is still the area at risk (Fig. 6.14). The medial papillary muscle tends to be at the apex of

these defects and the non-coronary aortic leaflet more closely related to the atrial margin. Often the septal leaflet of the tricuspid valve is cleft at the defect, an arrangement which may permit left ventricular-right atrial shunting. If the cleft requires surgical closure, it should be remembered that the penetrating bundle is located at its apex.

The final type of perimembranous defect extends mostly into the outlet of the right ventricle. The outlet septum is frequently hypoplastic (Fig. 6.15) or malaligned. The medial papillary muscle is on the right-hand margin and the conduction axis is more distant from the edge, being carried well down on the left ventricular septal surface. The non-coronary and right coronary aortic leaflets are much more closely related to the left-hand margin of the defect.

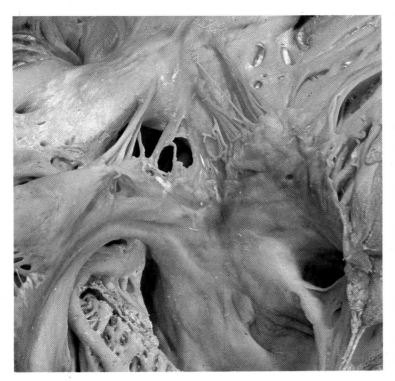

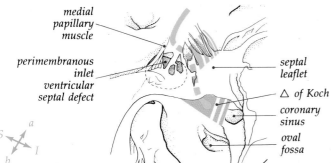

medial
papillary
muscle

perimembranous
inlet
ventricular
septal defect

septal
leaflet

△ of Koch

coronary
sinus

oval
fossa

Fig. 6.13 *Inlet perimembranous defect in surgical orientation.*

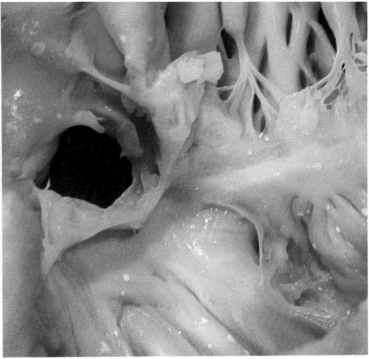

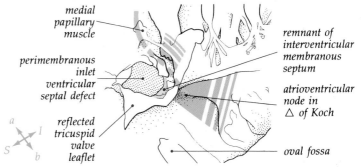

medial
papillary
muscle

perimembranous
inlet
ventricular
septal defect

reflected
tricuspid
valve
leaflet

remnant of
interventricular
membranous
septum

atrioventricular
node in
△ of Koch

oval fossa

Fig. 6.14 *Trabecular perimembranous defect in surgical orientation.*

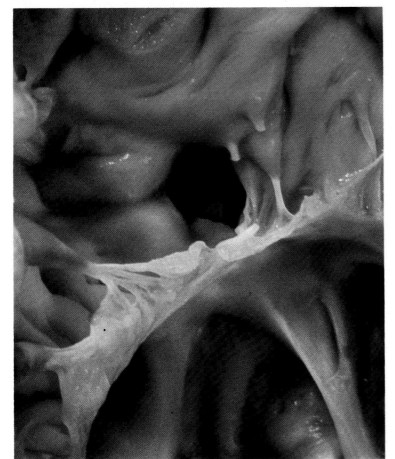

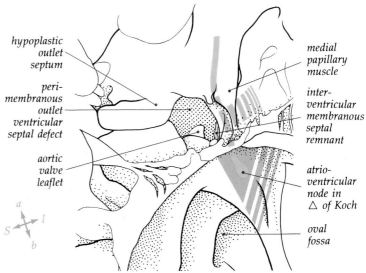

hypoplastic
outlet
septum

peri-
membranous
outlet
ventricular
septal defect

aortic
valve
leaflet

medial
papillary
muscle

inter-
ventricular
membranous
septal
remnant

atrio-
ventricular
node in
△ of Koch

oval
fossa

Fig. 6.15 *Outlet perimembranous defect with hypoplasia of the outlet septum, in surgical orientation. Compare the position of the medial papillary muscle with that in Figs. 6.13 & 6.14.*

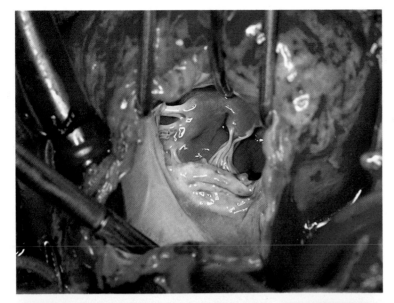

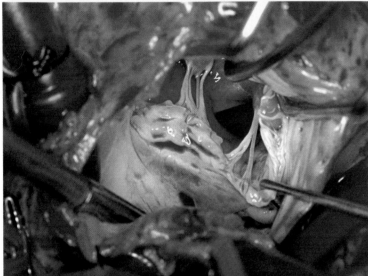

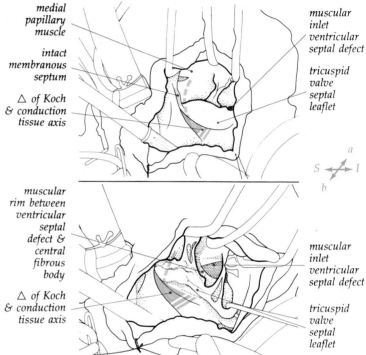

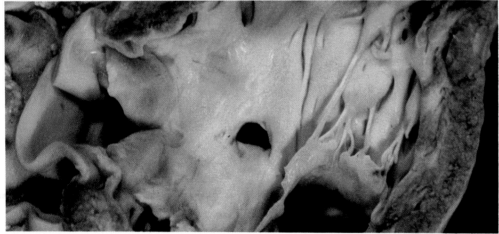

Fig. 6.16 *Muscular inlet ventricular septal defect: (upper) a broad muscle bundle separates the defect from the membranous septum. The conduction tissue courses to the left of the defect as the surgeon views it through the tricuspid valve; (lower) muscular rim of the defect beneath the retracted septal leaflet of the tricuspid valve.*

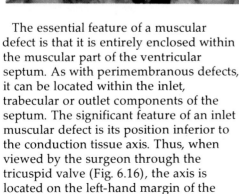

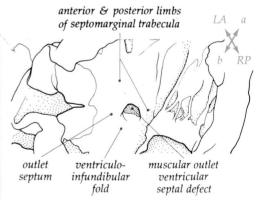

Fig. 6.17 *Muscular outlet defect, in surgical orientation.*

The essential feature of a muscular defect is that it is entirely enclosed within the muscular part of the ventricular septum. As with perimembranous defects, it can be located within the inlet, trabecular or outlet components of the septum. The significant feature of an inlet muscular defect is its position inferior to the conduction tissue axis. Thus, when viewed by the surgeon through the tricuspid valve (Fig. 6.16), the axis is located on the left-hand margin of the defect. The proximity of the axis to the edge depends upon how close the defect is to the intact membranous septal area. The muscular inlet defect also has a muscular bar separating the septal leaflet of the tricuspid valve from the mitral valve.

Defects in the trabecular part of the septum can be single and large, double and large, or multiple. They are unrelated to the proximal parts of the conduction tissue axis but may be related to ramifications of the distal bundle branches. The right ventricular aspect of these defects is frequently obscured by the coarse apical trabeculations. Indeed, multiple small defects may not be visible through a right ventriculotomy. In many instances, the openings can be more readily identified from the left ventricular aspect.

Muscular defects in the outlet septum are relatively rare in the normally connected heart and, when found, are usually small (Fig. 6.17). On initial inspection, the endocardium may appear to be heaped up at the edges to produce a

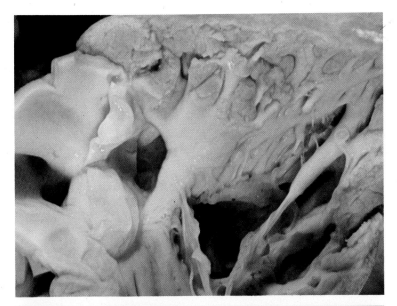

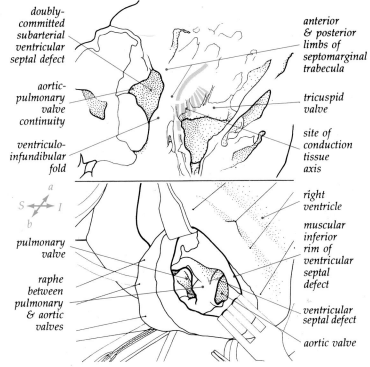

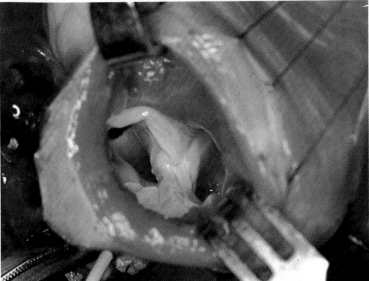

Fig. 6.18 *Doubly-committed subarterial defect with muscular posteroinferior rim: (upper) gross specimen; (lower) operative view of a similar defect.*

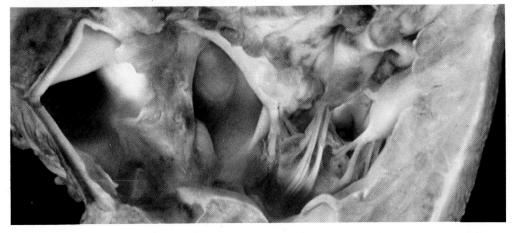

Fig. 6.19 *Doubly-committed subarterial defect which has extended, becoming perimembranous.*

fibrous rim. Nevertheless, close inspection will show that the posterior limb of the septomarginal trabecula is fused with the ventriculoinfundibular fold to form the posteroinferior rim of the defect. The fusion of these muscle bars separates the edge of the defect from the conduction tissue axis. The superior rim is the infundibular septum with the right coronary leaflet of the aortic valve attached to its left ventricular surface.

The final type of ventricular septal defect is the doubly-committed subarterial or 'supracristal' defect. The infundibular

septum is completely absent so that the facing leaflets of the aortic and pulmonary valves are in fibrous continuity and form the superior rim (Fig. 6.18). There may or may not be a firm fibrous raphe between the valves but, usually, sutures can be secured in the region of valvar fibrous continuity (Fig. 6.18, lower). The inferior rim of the defect is often similar to that found in the muscular outlet defect in that the posterior limb of the septomarginal trabecula fuses with the ventriculo-infundibular fold (Fig. 6.18). This muscular rim buttresses the conduction tissue axis

away from the edge of the defect. Occasionally a doubly-committed sub-arterial defect may extend to become perimembranous. The conduction axis is then much closer to the inferior corner of the defect (Fig. 6.19).

Although the above descriptions relate to ventricular septal defects in the normally connected heart, this typology and the guidance it gives to the conduction tissues are also valid for hearts with atrioventricular concordance but abnormal ventriculoarterial connexions (see Chapter 7, iii, v & vi).

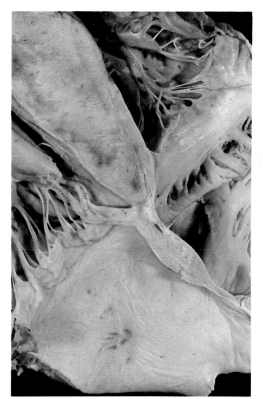
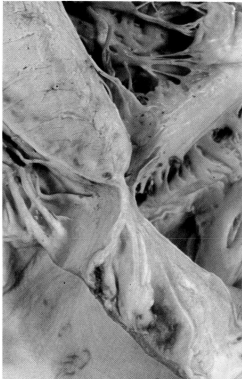
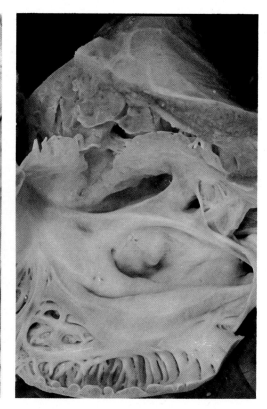

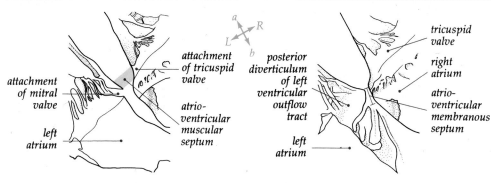

Fig. 6.20 *Long-axis sections at right angles to the septum showing (left) muscular and (right) membranous atrioventricular septal structures, in surgical orientation.*

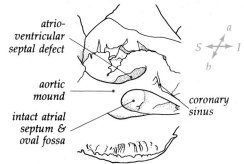

Fig. 6.21 *Opened right atrioventricular junction of a so-called 'partial endocardial cushion defect' or 'ostium primum atrial septal defect', which is actually an atrioventricular septal defect, in surgical orientation. The atrial septum is normally formed and the oval fossa is intact.*

iii. Atrioventricular septal defects

'Atrioventricular septal defect' is, we believe, the most suitable collective term for the anomalies variously described, amongst others, as 'endocardial cushion defects' and 'persistent atrioventricular canal'. This is because, in anatomic terms, the malformations are primarily due to absence of the usual atrioventricular septal structures.

In the normal heart there is an atrioventricular membranous septum (Fig. 6.20, right) and an atrioventricular muscular septum (Fig. 6.20, left). The former exists because the tricuspid valve attachment to the septum is further towards the apex than the septal attachment of the mitral valve. A defect at the site of these structures (Fig. 6.21) characterizes 'endocardial cushion defects', whether of complete, partial or intermediate type (*Van Mierop, 1970; Becker & Anderson, 1982*).

Because of the lack of these atrioventricular septal structures, there is no septal atrioventricular junction. Instead, the opposing arches formed by the leading edges of the atrial and ventricular septa (the latter usually covered by the atrioventricular valve leaflets) meet at the anterior and posterior margins of a common atrioventricular junction. This anatomy determines the anomalous disposition of the atrioventricular conduction axis. The triangle of Koch is well formed in the edge of the arch of the atrial septum but, because of the septal defect, it has no contact with the ventricular myocardium. Thus, the atrioventricular node is displaced posteriorly, lying in a nodal triangle whose margins, as seen by the surgeon, are the right-hand edge of the atrial septum and the attachment of the atrioventricular valve leaflet (Fig. 6.22). The bundle penetrates through the apex

of this triangle to run on the crest of the ventricular septum, covered by the inferior bridging leaflet of the valve (see below).

The base of this nodal triangle is the coronary sinus. The length of its vertex is pertinent to surgical closure. Ideally the surgeon wishes to place his patch so as to leave the coronary sinus draining to the systemic venous atrium. In the heart in Fig. 6.22 the sizeable post-Eustachian sinus would make this feasible; but in other hearts, the coronary sinus lies much closer to the apex of the nodal triangle and the length of the vertex is such that placement of a suture line through it would seriously endanger the node. In those cases it would seem prudent to place the patch so that the coronary sinus drains to the pulmonary venous atrium.

The feature which distinguishes the various forms of atrioventricular septal defects is the morphology of the

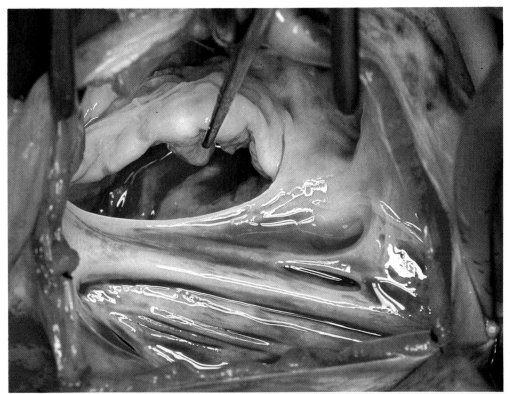

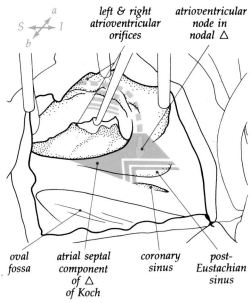

Fig. 6.22 *Operative view of atrioventricular septal defect with separate valve orifices ('ostium primum atrial septal defect'). The atrioventricular septal part of the triangle of Koch is missing, thereby displacing the conduction axis into the nodal triangle.*

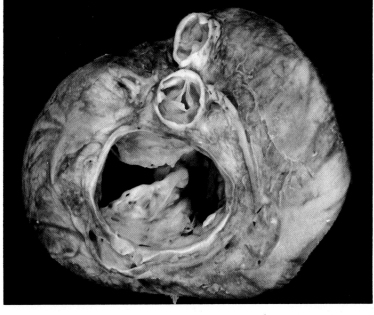

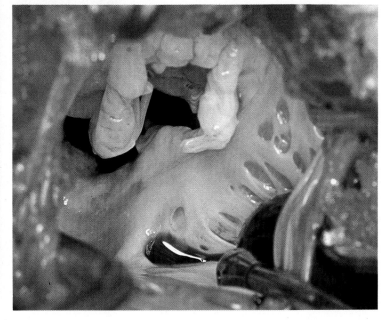

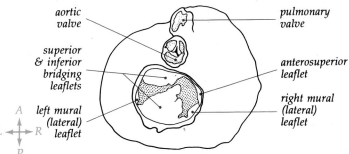

Fig. 6.23 *Short-axis view from above of common atrioventricular junction of an atrioventricular septal defect with common orifice. The valve has five leaflets.*

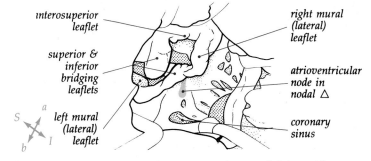

Fig. 6.24 *Operative view of atrioventricular septal defect with common atrioventricular valve orifice ('complete defect'). The position of the atrioventricular node in the nodal triangle is indicated.*

atrioventricular valve leaflets and their relationship to the ventricular septum (*Van Mierop, 1970*). In any atrioventricular septal defect, the valve is basically a common valve with five leaflets. This is most readily seen in a defect with a common valve orifice (Figs. 6.23 & 6.24). Two of the leaflets straddle the ventricular septum and are tethered in both ventricles; these are the superior and inferior bridging leaflets. Two leaflets are entirely contained within the right ventricle and are the anterosuperior and mural (lateral) leaflets. The final leaflet is contained within the left ventricle and is also a mural leaflet.

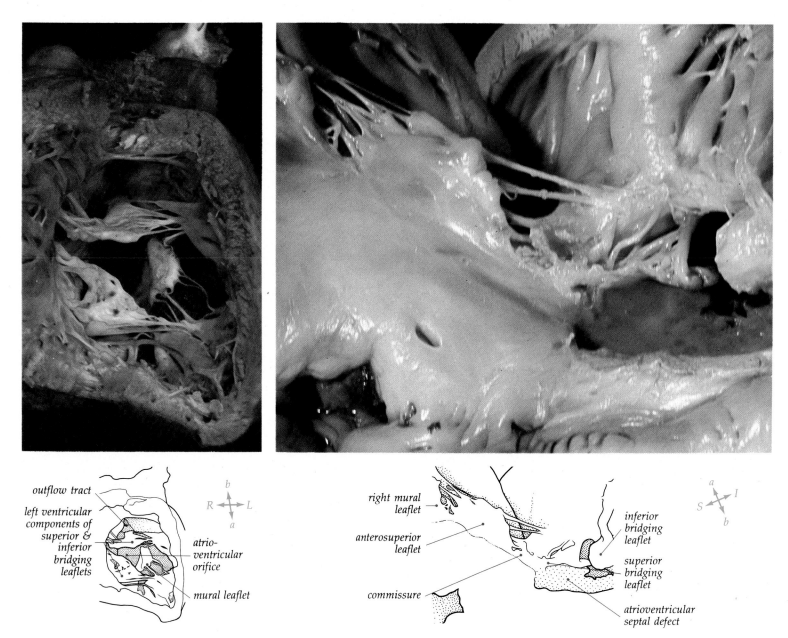

Fig. 6.25 *Trifoliate left atrioventricular valve in atrioventricular septal defect, in anatomical orientation.*

Fig. 6.26 *Commissure between the superior bridging leaflet and the right anterosuperior leaflet in a so-called 'Rastelli type A' anomaly, in surgical orientation.*

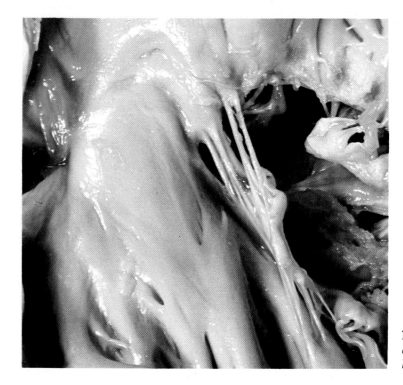

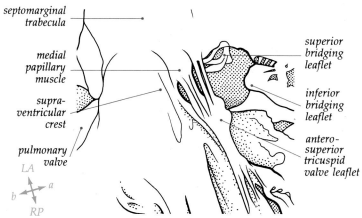

Fig. 6.27 *Outlet viewed from the right ventricular apex of the commissure between the superior bridging leaflet and the anterosuperior leaflet, supported by the medial papillary muscle.*

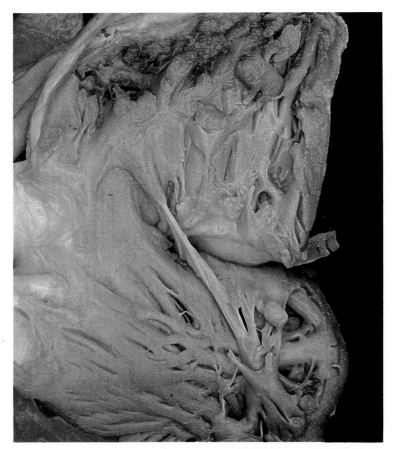

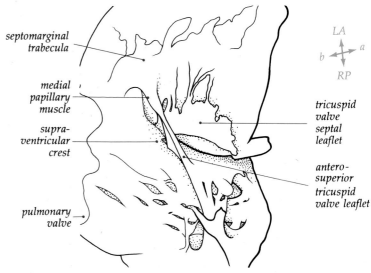

septomarginal trabecula

medial papillary muscle

supra-ventricular crest

pulmonary valve

tricuspid valve septal leaflet

antero-superior tricuspid valve leaflet

LA
b   a
RP

Fig. 6.28 *Normal heart viewed as in Fig. 6.27 showing similar position of the medial papillary muscle.*

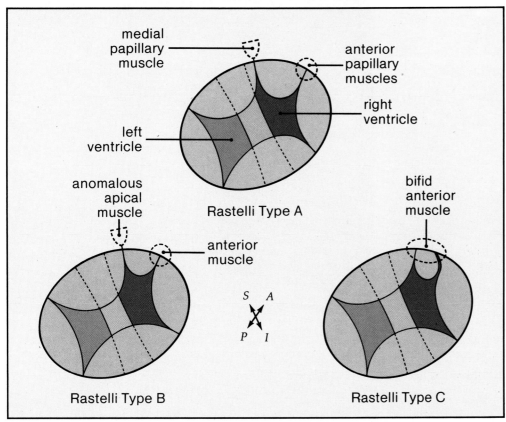

medial papillary muscle

anterior papillary muscles

right ventricle

left ventricle

Rastelli Type A

anomalous apical muscle

anterior muscle

Rastelli Type B

bifid anterior muscle

S   A
P   I

Rastelli Type C

Fig. 6.29 *Spectrum of degree of bridging of the superior bridging leaflet which underscores the Rastelli classification of atrioventricular septal defect with common orifice.*

Although the two right ventricular leaflets are comparable to similar leaflets seen in the normal heart, the left ventricular side of a common atrioventricular valve bears scant resemblance to a normal mitral valve. The commissures and papillary muscles of the normal mitral valve are situated posteroseptally and anterolaterally within the orifice, producing an extensive mural leaflet subdivided into its characteristic scallops (see Fig. 2.20). In atrioventricular septal defects, the left ventricular papillary muscles are deviated laterally so that the mural leaflet is relatively insignificant. The left orifice is, in effect, guarded by a trifoliate valve comprising the small mural leaflet and the left ventricular components of the superior and inferior bridging leaflets (Fig. 6.25).

Traditional thought (*Rastelli, Kirklin & Titus, 1966*) is that the valve morphology in the presence of a common orifice consists of a four-leaflet valve with a cleft in the 'common anterior leaflet'. In fact, close examination of this 'cleft' (Fig. 6.26) will show that, on the infundibular aspect, it is supported by the medial papillary muscle of the right ventricle (Fig. 6.27). When seen from the outflow tract, it is virtually indistinguishable from the anteroseptal commissure of a normal tricuspid valve (Fig. 6.28). This is, therefore, minimal bridging of the superior leaflet into the right ventricle with the commissure between it and the anterosuperior leaflet supported by the medial papillary muscle. The variability noted by Rastelli et al. (1966) is readily explained by increased commitment of the superior bridging leaflet to the right ventricle, with concomitant diminution in size of the anterosuperior leaflet and movement of the papillary muscle supporting the commissure towards the right ventricular apex (*Piccoli et al., 1979; Fig. 6.29*). A further difference between the hearts at either end of this spectrum is that with minimal bridging the superior bridging leaflet is tethered to the crest of the septum whereas with extreme bridging the leaflet tends to be free-floating. Tethering of the bridging leaflets to the septum accounts for much of the remaining variability in atrioventricular septal defects.

6.13

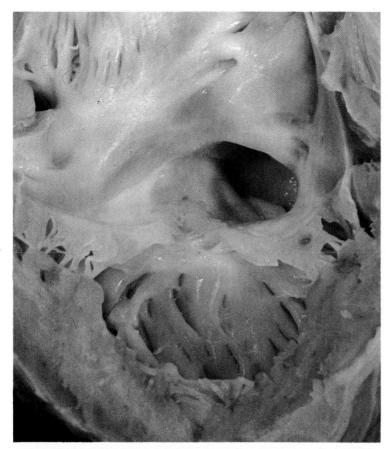

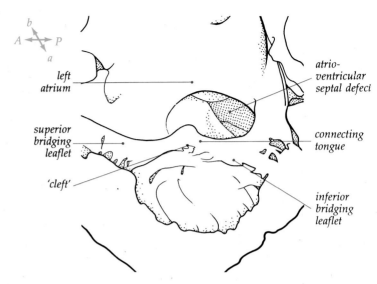

Fig. 6.30 *Gap between facing surfaces of left ventricular components of bridging leaflets in an ostium primum atrial septal defect which is usually referred to as a 'cleft', in anatomical orientation. It is not comparable to the cleft which can exist in the aortic leaflet of the normal mitral valve (see Fig. 6.41).*

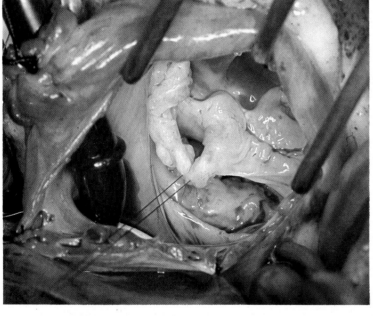

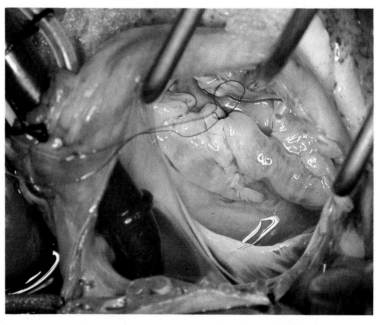

Fig. 6.31 *Operative view showing a suture closing the gap between bridging leaflets in an ostium primum atrial septal defect. Prior to repair, the gap allowed left ventricular–right atrial shunting.*

Fig. 6.32 *Operative view of the gap between bridging leaflets after closure to prevent regurgitation. The resultant valve does not resemble a normal mitral valve.*

In the so-called 'partial' atrioventricular septal defect, also referred to as the 'ostium primum atrial septal defect', the overall valve morphology is comparable to that seen in the variant with common valve orifice ('complete' defect). However, the two bridging leaflets in the partial defect are firmly fused to the ventricular septum (the atrioventricular septum being absent) and are joined to each other by a connecting tongue which is adherent to the septal crest (Fig. 6.30). Thus, the essence of the partial form is the separate right and left valve orifices. The so-called 'cleft' in the 'mitral' valve of an ostium

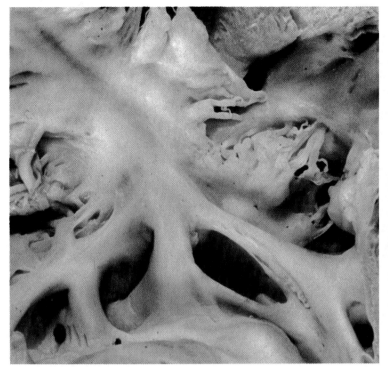

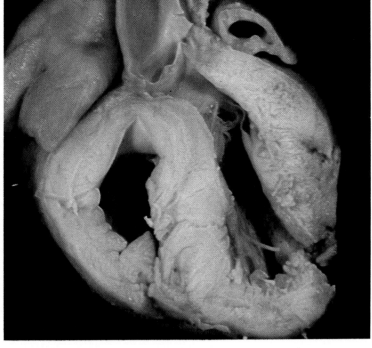

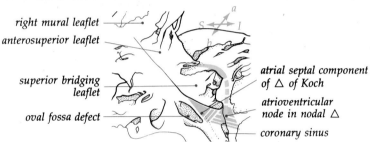

right mural leaflet

anterosuperior leaflet

superior bridging leaflet

oval fossa defect

atrial septal component of △ of Koch

atrioventricular node in nodal △

coronary sinus

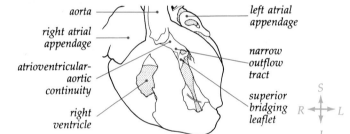

aorta

right atrial appendage

atrioventricular-aortic continuity

right ventricle

left atrial appendage

narrow outflow tract

superior bridging leaflet

Fig. 6.33 *Right ventricular aspect of an atrioventricular septal defect with common orifice, in surgical orientation. The course of the conduction tissue axis is shown.*

Fig. 6.34 *Long-axis section at right angles to the septum through the outflow tract in atrioventricular septal defect showing its intrinsic narrowness.*

primum atrial septal defect is the space between the left ventricular components of the superior and inferior bridging leaflets. This 'cleft' is not comparable to the cleft in the aortic leaflet of the normal mitral valve. If surgical repair of this 'cleft' is required (Fig. 6.31), one should not make the mistake of attempting to recreate a leaflet comparable to the aortic leaflet of the mitral valve (Fig. 6.32).

There are various ways of categorizing intermediate forms of atrioventricular septal defect. The presence of a connecting tongue (as described above) clearly divides the common junction into left and right components. Some define intermediate forms where there are two separate orifices in the common junction but, because the leaflets are not fused to the ventricular septal crest, there are coexisting interventricular communications (*Brandt et al., 1972*). Others define intermediate forms where the two bridging leaflets are firmly fused to the septum but with no connecting tongue so that, although presenting surgically as an 'ostium primum', there is in fact a common atrioventricular orifice (*Wakai & Edwards, 1956*). Still others have combined these two approaches to produce a classification of bewildering complexity

(*Bharati et al., 1980*). We see no need for such complex classifications as the variability can be readily understood on the basis of the relationships of the bridging leaflets to each other and to the ventricular septum. The variability is best described in terms of a common orifice or separate right and left valve orifices, together with the presence or absence of an interventricular communication.

It is evident from our discussion that the basic morphology of the ventricular septum is comparable in all atrioventricular septal defects and determines the disposition of the ventricular conduction pathways. Although the hallmark of the malformation is absence of the atrioventricular muscular and membranous septal structures, there is also hypoplasia to a greater or lesser extent of the muscular ventricular septum. The degree of hypoplasia of the inlet septum determines how much the septum appears to be 'scooped out'. The non-branching bundle runs down the crest of this part of the septum and is covered by the inferior bridging leaflet. Often, the inferior leaflet itself is divided by a midline raphe immediately above the vulnerable non-branching bundle.

The branching bundle is found astride

the midportion of the septal crest, usually covered by the connecting tongue in partial defects but sometimes exposed in the presence of a common orifice and free-floating leaflets. The right bundle branch then runs towards the medial papillary muscle. Anterior to this point the septum is devoid of conduction tissue (Fig. 6.33).

Although not readily evident to the surgeon during operation, the left ventricular outflow tract in atrioventricular septal defects is intrinsically narrow (Fig. 6.34). Thus, it is vulnerable to obstruction either by naturally occurring lesions (*Piccoli et al., 1982*) or by injudicious placement of a left atrioventricular valve prosthesis. If a prosthesis must be employed, the anatomy dictates insertion of a low-profile model.

Finally, there is variability in the commitment of the common atrioventricular junction to the ventricular mass. Usually it is shared equally, giving the balanced form; but if the orifice favours one ventricle (right or left ventricular dominance; *Bharati & Lev, 1973*), the other ventricle is often severely hypoplastic. This can have a major influence on the outcome of surgery and should always be assessed preoperatively.

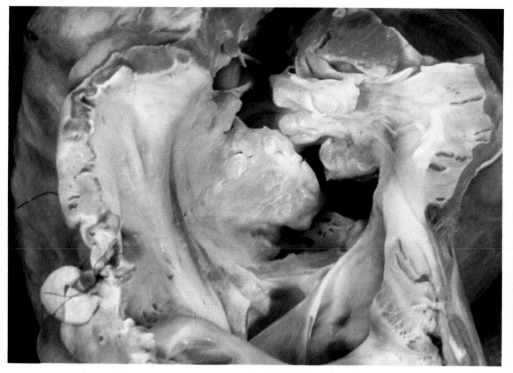

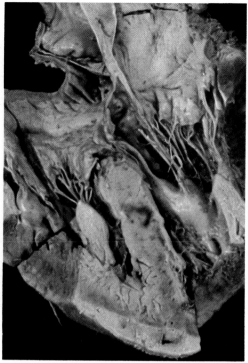

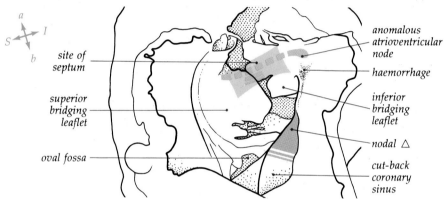

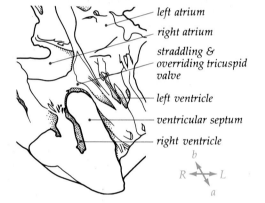

Fig. 6.35 *Right inlet aspect of atrioventricular septal defect with left ventricular dominance. The gross malalignment between atrial and ventricular septa has placed the atrioventricular node in an anomalous position; compare with Fig. 6.38.*

Fig. 6.36 *Long-axis 'four-chamber' view of a straddling and overriding right atrioventricular valve.*

Recently we studied a case of left ventricular dominance in which the morphology underscoring the ventricular disproportion was particularly significant. There was malalignment between the atrial septum, which was poorly formed in the presence of a persistent left superior caval vein draining to the coronary sinus, and the inlet part of the ventricular septum (Fig. 6.35). This produced an arrangement analogous to straddling of the tricuspid valve (see below). The malaligned atrial and ventricular septa meant that the connecting atrioventricular node was no longer at the apex of the nodal triangle. Instead, it was where the ventricular septum met the atrioventricular junction and had been traumatized during placement of the atrial patch (*Pillai et al., 1984*). This arrangement should be identified preoperatively since it can be exceedingly difficult to recognize during operation. It should certainly be considered as a possible cause for concern in all cases of atrioventricular septal defect with left ventricular dominance.

iv. Atrioventricular valve malformations

The pathological lesions which affect atrioventricular valves, both acquired and congenital, are legion and not all are amenable to surgical repair. Those interested in the overall pathology are referred to recent reviews (*Becker & Anderson, 1981; Becker, 1983*); we concentrate here on features of immediate surgical relevance.

The anatomy of atrioventricular valves themselves indicates that problems may be encountered in the annulus, in the leaflets or in the tension apparatus. Sometimes the valve and the atrio-ventricular connexion are totally absent (valve 'atresia'; see Chapter 7). The lesions considered in this section can affect either tricuspid or mitral valves but, because the tricuspid valve usually functions in a low pressure environment, the lesions are more frequently manifest in the mitral valve. We will deal with each lesion in turn, indicating its proclivity towards one or the other valve.

Of considerable surgical significance is overriding of the valve annulus. Almost always this is associated with straddling of the tension apparatus (Fig. 6.36). Although the site of insertion of the tension apparatus across the septum determines the surgical options, the override is also important. Overriding usually indicates septal malalignment with its consequential conduction tissue disposition. Straddling and overriding can affect either valve and occur in various chamber combinations. (For straddling in the setting of double inlet ventricle and atrioventricular discordance, see Chapter 7). Here we are concerned with straddling valves with atrioventricular concordance.

When the mitral valve straddles an anterior ventricular septal defect with the inlet septum normally related to the crux (Fig. 6.37), the conduction tissue is normally disposed. Usually the antero-lateral papillary muscle of the mitral valve is attached within the right ventricle and arises from the septomarginal trabecula alongside, but separate from, the anterior

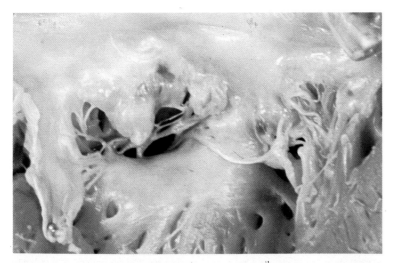

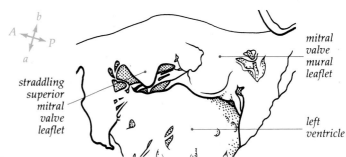

Fig. 6.37 *Straddling mitral valve viewed from the left ventricular aspect, in anatomical orientation.*

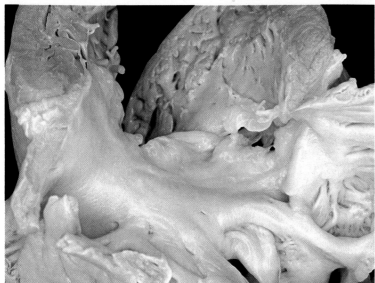

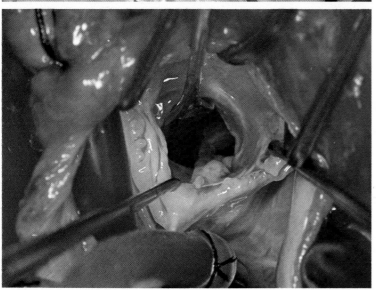

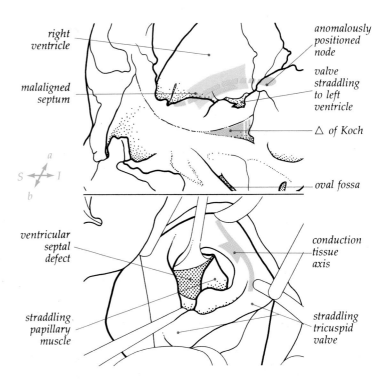

Fig. 6.38 *Straddling tricuspid valve: (upper) view through right atrioventricular junction to show the septal malalignment and anomalous conduction tissue disposition; compare with Fig. 6.35; (lower) operative view. Upper by courtesy of Dr. J.R. Zuberbuhler.*

papillary muscle of the tricuspid valve. This arrangement, often seen with either complete transposition or double outlet right ventricle with subpulmonary defect, can seriously compromise surgical repair.

Straddling of the tricuspid valve is found more frequently with isolated ventricular septal defects (Fig. 6.38, lower) or tetralogy, but it may also exist with abnormal ventriculoarterial connexions (Fig. 6.38, upper). The salient feature is that the ventricular septum does not extend to the crux and the defect is due to malalignment in the inlet ventricular component. The conduction tissue originates not from the normal atrioventricular node but from an anomalous node in the posterolateral margin of the right atrioventricular junction (Fig. 6.38) and runs back onto the septal crest. Usually the septal leaflet is tethered to the enlarged posteromedial papillary muscle of the mitral valve. A 'mini-septation' procedure is often necessary for complete ventricular repair, which carries a high risk of producing heart block (*Pacifico, Soto & Bargeron,*

1979). Alternative approaches have been discussed by McGoon et al. (1981).

Dilatation of the annulus of the valve occurs almost exclusively as an acquired lesion. A dilated mitral annulus is most frequently secondary to myocarditis. When surgical narrowing of the orifice is indicated, often it can be accomplished using various annuloplasty techniques without resorting to valve replacement. Dilatation of the tricuspid annulus is seen most frequently as a result of right heart failure.

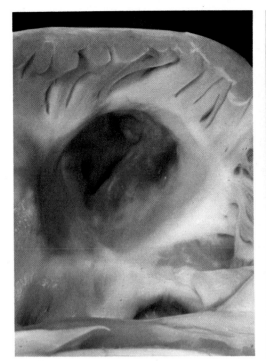

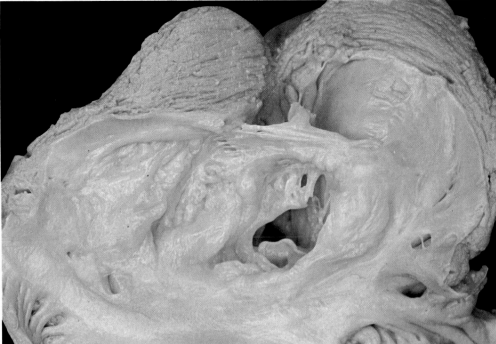

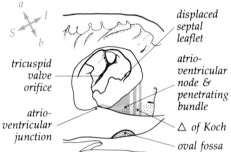

Fig. 6.39 *Right atrioventricular junction in Ebstein's malformation viewed from the atrial aspect. The triangle of Koch is still the guide to the conduction axis.*

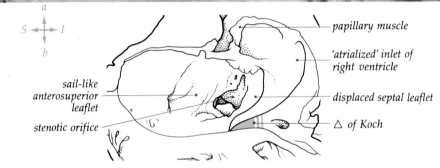

Fig. 6.40 *Opened tricuspid orifice of heart with Ebstein's malformation, in surgical orientation. By courtesy of Dr. J. R. Zuberbuhler.*

Of more significance surgically is the dilatation which accompanies Ebstein's malformation. The crucial feature of this anomaly is displacement of the attachment of the septal and mural valve leaflets towards the junction of the ventricular inlet and trabecular components (Fig. 6.39). The anterosuperior leaflet is less affected but may sometimes be attached across the inlet-trabecular junction as a curtain, acutely restricting antegrade flow into the pulmonary trunk (Fig. 6.40). In the most severe form, the anterosuperior leaflet completely blocks this junction, producing an imperforate Ebstein's malformation which presents as tricuspid atresia (see Chapter 7, ii).

Ebstein's malformation requires surgical treatment when there is significant dilatation of the true atrioventricular annulus, and the wall of the right ventricular inlet component is both dilated and thinned. Reparative operations require suture placement in the area of thinning and particular care should be taken to avoid the right coronary artery and its branches. In the septal area the triangle of Koch remains the guide to the atrioventricular conduction axis (see Figs. 6.39 & 4.4). Ebstein's malformation

involving the left-sided morphologically tricuspid valve in congenitally corrected transposition is discussed in Chapter 7, iv, but it should be remembered that, rarely, an Ebstein-like lesion can involve the normally located morphologically mitral valve (*Ruschaupt, Bharati & Lev, 1976*).

Malformations of the valve leaflets can be summarized in terms of dysplasia, prolapse and clefts. The morphology of the dysplastic process is thickening and 'heaping up' of the valve leaflet, usually with obliteration of the interchordal spaces. A dysplastic valve may pose a significant surgical problem. It is frequently seen with outflow tract atresia and as an integral part of Ebstein's anomaly. Isolated dysplasia is exceedingly rare.

Prolapse of valve leaflets occurs more frequently and is usually associated with deficiency of the tension apparatus. It can be repaired by valve replacement or by various valvuloplasty techniques, including chordal shortening.

The isolated cleft can be repaired by reconstituting its edges. Isolated clefts of the aortic leaflet of the mitral valve should be distinguished from so-called 'clefts' in atrioventricular septal defects (Fig. 6.41;

compare with Fig. 6.30).

We have already discussed some of the abnormalities of the tension apparatus that accompany annular or leaflet malformations, such as straddling papillary muscles. The so-called 'parachute' deformity is the most worrisome lesion of the tension apparatus, apart from exceptionally rare anomalies such as arcade lesions (*Layman & Edwards, 1967*). There is some confusion about the definition of a 'parachute' valve. Some would define it as fusion of the papillary muscle groups so that all the chords insert into a common muscle mass (*Rosenquist, 1974*). Others (*Ruckman & Van Praagh, 1978*), following the original description of Shone et al. (1963), define a parachute lesion of the mitral valve as absence or gross hypoplasia of one commissure with absence of its supporting papillary muscle. Either way, surgical reconstruction is difficult and valve replacement is likely to be necessary. Parachute deformity of the mitral valve may be further complicated by other lesions such as supravalvular left atrial stenosing ring and coarctation of the aorta. Parachute malformation of the tricuspid valve can occur but is rarely of clinical significance.

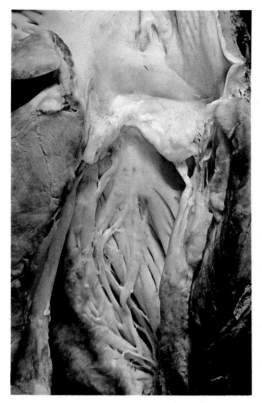

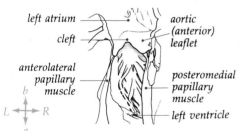

Fig. 6.41 *Isolated cleft in aortic leaflet of an otherwise normal mitral valve, in anatomical orientation. Compare with the 'cleft' in Fig. 6.30. By courtesy of Prof. A. E. Becker.*

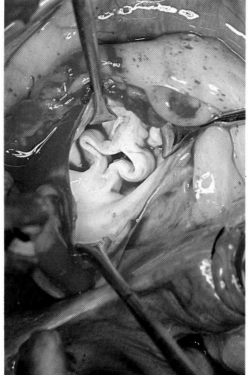

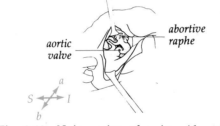

Fig. 6.42 *Unicommissural, unicuspid aortic valve as seen during operation.*

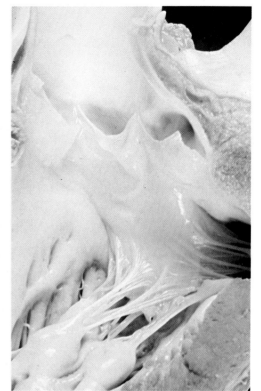

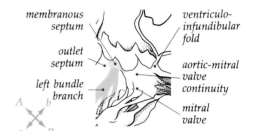

Fig. 6.43 *Normal left ventricular outflow tract and the course of the left bundle branch, in anatomical orientation.*

v. Arterial valve and outflow tract malformations

In this section we describe the surgical aspects of ventricular outflow tract obstruction, valvular stenosis and outflow tract atresia. In the normally connected heart, obstruction in the left ventricular outflow tract produces subaortic stenosis. It must be remembered that the same anatomic lesions will produce sub-pulmonary obstruction in the patient with complete transposition. Similarly, right ventricular outflow tract obstruction produces subpulmonary obstruction in the normally connected heart but subaortic stenosis in complete trans-position. When both outflow tracts are connected to the same ventricular chamber, the anatomical problems are more discrete. These are considered separately in Chapter 7, v.

Aortic valve stenosis can be discussed at valvular, subvalvular and supravalvular levels. Aortic regurgitation is ultimately a valvular problem and the perivalvular anatomy is often of great importance. Valvular aortic stenosis may occur with unicuspid, bicuspid, tricuspid and, rarely, even quadricuspid valves. Dysplastic

lesions are also seen in the aortic valve but only rarely can surgery provide the answer to this problem. The unicuspid valve usually has one or two abortive commissural raphes (Fig. 6.42). Little can be done other than an attempt to open the valve as much as possible, short of producing severe regurgitation. Attempts to open the rudimentary raphe invariably result in valve prolapse and regurgitation.

A bicuspid valve is most frequently seen in the adult patient. Perhaps this is because a bicuspid valve may not be intrinsically stenotic. Usually it is only after the effects of time and turbulence that these valves become manifestly obstructive. If the valvular topology has not been totally obscured by calcific deposits, a bicuspid valve seen at operation will take one of two forms. Occasionally the two leaflets are of equal size, the commissures bisecting the aortic root. This type is frequently found in patients with coarctation of the aorta. In the other form, the cusps are unequal with the large, or conjoined, cusp almost always exhibiting an eccentrically-placed raphe. The 'sinus' of the conjoined cusp usually gives rise to both coronary arteries from an anterior

position. If these valves are seen before they become rigid and distorted by calcification, some relief from the stenosis can be obtained by careful enlargement of the single commissure.

Aortic stenosis does occur in patients with three valve leaflets, but this is rather rare. A possible cause of such stenoses is the unequal size of the cusps in the normal aortic valve which, coupled with the high pressure flow in the aortic root, may lead to the development of calcification and stenosis in the elderly (*Vollebergh & Becker, 1977*).

Subvalvular stenosis may be fibrous, fibromuscular or muscular as the left ventricular outflow tract is partly muscular and partly fibrous. The muscular portion comprises the ventriculo-infundibular fold anterolaterally, the outlet septum anteriorly and the upper edge of the trabecular septum medially. The fibrous part comprises the central fibrous body, the area of aortic-mitral continuity and the left fibrous trigone (Fig. 6.43). Also, subvalvular stenoses may be either fixed or dynamic in nature.

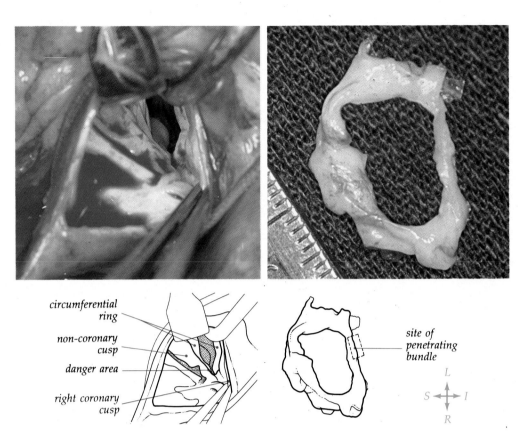

circumferential ring

non-coronary cusp

danger area

right coronary cusp

site of penetrating bundle

L

S ← I

R

Fig. 6.44 *Discrete circumferential subaortic membrane seen (left) through the aortic valve and (right) in isolation after removal.*

Of the fixed variety, a subvalvular fibrous 'diaphragm' is perhaps most easily approached surgically. Though it appears circular when viewed through the usually normal aortic valve, and indeed it can be circular (Fig. 6.44), this is not always the case. Sometimes a relatively thin shelf of tissue runs from beneath the non-coronary cusp of the aortic valve, over the site of the penetrating bundle to the septal musculature, finally coursing over the ventriculoinfundibular fold to involve the aortic leaflet of the mitral valve (Fig. 6.45). If the operation is performed prudently (*McKay & Ross, 1982*), a circumferential lesion can be completely removed (Fig. 6.44, right), taking particular care where the diaphragm intimately overlies the conduction tissues. Too vigorous an attack on the side of the mitral valve may lead to detachment of that structure.

In cases where complete removal proves difficult, interruption of the fibrous diaphragm in the safe area over the ventriculoinfundibular fold will result in a safe and satisfactory relief of the stenosis. The same rules apply when resecting the fibromuscular tunnel form of aortic stenosis, although surgical correction may be less successful since this lesion extends farther into the left ventricle, making its obstruction more difficult to interrupt.

A rather rare form of fixed subaortic obstruction has been reported by Moulaert and Oppenheimer-Dekker (1976), namely hypertrophy of the usually inconspicuous anterolateral muscle bundle. This muscle runs down the outflow tract

from the ventriculoinfundibular fold to the ventricular septum. In its course over the parietal wall it would not be expected to involve the conduction tissues.

Anomalous attachment of the mitral valve can cause fixed obstruction, as can a deviated infundibular septum. The former is usually seen with atrioventricular septal defect, and the latter occurs only, but not always, with ventricular septal defect.

The final fixed type of subaortic obstruction is produced by so-called 'tissue tags'. These herniate from any adjacent fibrous tissue structure but are exceedingly rare as an isolated lesion in the normally connected heart (*Anderson, Lenox & Zuberbuhler, 1983*). They can produce significant left ventricular outflow tract obstruction in hearts with an atrioventricular septal defect or complete transposition.

Dynamic subvalvular obstruction is a result of thickening of the septal musculature abutting the aortic leaflet of the mitral valve during ventricular systole. This usually creates a ridge of thickened endocardium easily seen through the aortic valve. If an operation becomes necessary, resection of this muscle bundle, as advocated by Morrow et al. (1959), offers satisfactory relief of the obstruction. Again the surgeon must scrupulously avoid the conduction tissue as it emerges beneath the commissure between the right and non-coronary cusps and descends on the interventricular septum.

Supravalvular aortic stenosis is said to occur as one of three types: an hourglass, a membranous and a more diffuse tubular

deformity (*Edwards, 1965*). All forms are rare and, fortunately, the severe tubular type is extremely unusual. Two problems are shared by all three varieties because of narrowing of the aorta at the aortic bar, which is the junction of the aortic root and ascending aorta. Firstly, the aortic root, which usually contains the coronary arteries, is converted into a high pressure zone in which the arteries provide the only run-off other than through the distal stenosis. This produces marked dilatation of the coronary arteries. Secondly, the circumferential narrowing at the aortic bar tends to tether the three aortic cusps in such a way that it is rarely enough to perform a simple 'aortoplasty' whereby the ring is interrupted by enlarging one sinus with a patch. As Doty, Polansky & Jenson (1977) have observed, at least two, and sometimes all three, sinuses must be opened up to allow adequate relief of this obstruction.

Aortic valvular insufficiency may be due to congenital malformation of the valve, its supporting structures or both, or it may be secondary to an infectious process in the aortic root or to 'degenerative' disease. Occasionally, aortic insufficiency may be due to trauma. Its frequent association with the doubly-committed subarterial 'supracristal' ventricular septal defect (*Van Praagh & McNamara, 1968*) suggests that deficiency in the valvular support structure plays some role in these problems. Aortic valve prolapse and insufficiency may occur with other types of ventricular septal defect or with none at all, the latter situation being associated usually with a bicuspid aortic valve.

The critical importance of the anatomy of this region is perhaps best demonstrated by the problems exhibited by patients with aortic valve endocarditis. Because the aortic valve is the 'keystone' to all the other valves and chambers of the heart, an eroding abscess in the aortic root may lead to formation of a fistula involving any of these adjacent structures. Thus, the patient may present with findings of left heart failure, left-to-right shunting, complete heart block or any combination of these, in addition to the usual signs of sepsis. Surgical management clearly requires a detailed knowledge of this area since one may be faced with virtual disruption of the ventriculoarterial connexion (*Frantz, Murray & Wilcox, 1980*). A very similar problem can occur when the aortic root, or the fibrous 'coronet' (see Fig. 2.21), is severely damaged by aortic root dissection or marked degeneration of its fibrous structure.

As with aortic stenosis, pulmonary stenosis can occur at the valvular, supravalvular or subvalvular levels. The latter is discussed in detail in association with tetralogy of Fallot (see below). Pulmonary valve dysplasia is most often seen as marked distortion and thickening of the valve, although three 'leaflets' can

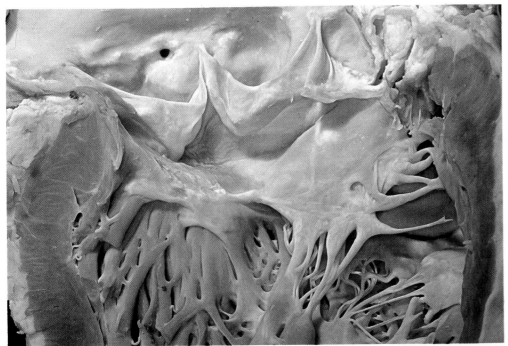

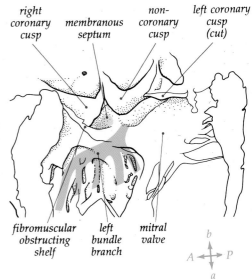

right coronary cusp — membranous septum — non-coronary cusp — left coronary cusp (cut)

fibromuscular obstructing shelf — left bundle branch — mitral valve

b
A ←→ P
a

Fig. 6.45 *Fixed subaortic diaphragm and position of the left bundle branch, in anatomical orientation. By courtesy of Prof. A. E. Becker.*

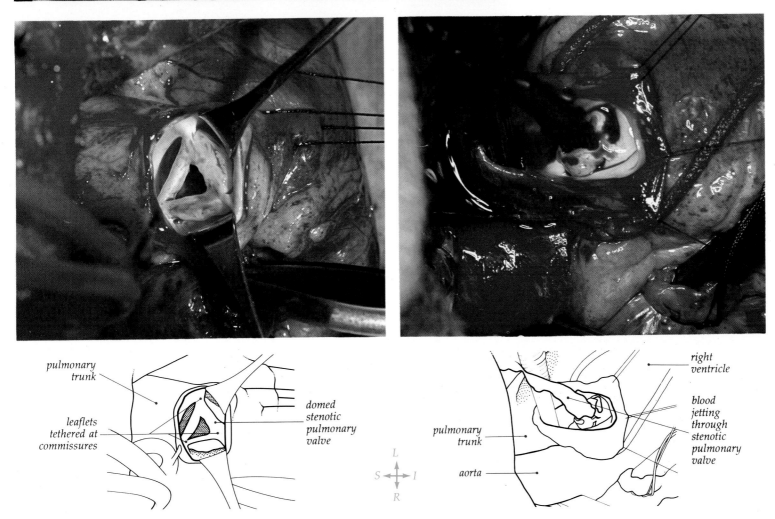

pulmonary trunk

leaflets tethered at commissures

domed stenotic pulmonary valve

L
S ←→ I
R

right ventricle

blood jetting through stenotic pulmonary valve

pulmonary trunk

aorta

Fig. 6.46 *Operative view of dome-shaped and stenotic pulmonary valve with three fused commissures.*

Fig. 6.47 *Streaming of blood through a stenotic pulmonary valve.*

sometimes be recognized. It can be associated with insufficiency as well as stenosis.

Isolated pulmonary stenosis is often found in the form of a dome-shaped valve with three well developed but fused commissures (Fig. 6.46). In some cases, the valve appears to be attached to the wall of the pulmonary artery along the commissural lines, leaving only a restricted opening to the valve (Fig. 6.47) and a narrowed pulmonary arterial root. These attachments can be dissected from the arterial wall and incised, resulting in a more satisfactory relief of the obstruction. The effectiveness of surgery is best measured six to nine months after operation, since significant secondary obstruction at the subvalvular level may maintain a pressure gradient across the outflow tract. This muscular hypertrophy will almost always regress with time (*Gilbert, Morrow & Talbert, 1963*).

Supravalvular stenosis usually takes the

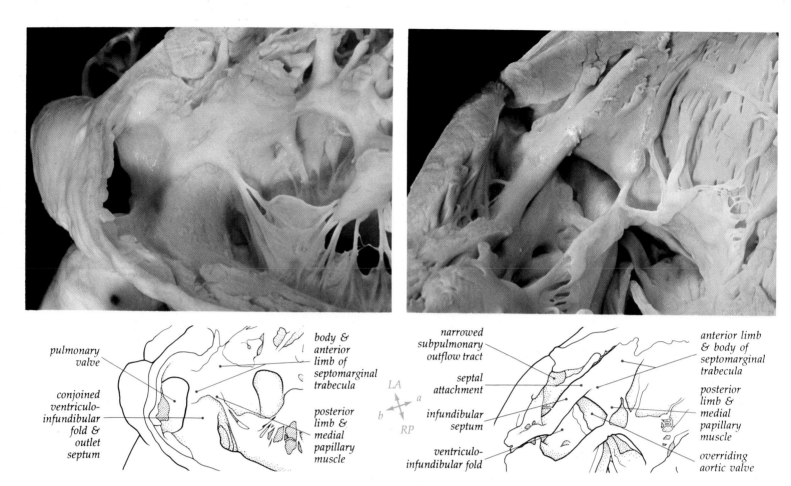

Fig. 6.48 *Right ventricular outflow tract of normal heart, in surgical orientation.*

pulmonary valve

conjoined ventriculo-infundibular fold & outlet septum

body & anterior limb of septomarginal trabecula

posterior limb & medial papillary muscle

Fig. 6.49 *Typical features of tetralogy of Fallot, seen by looking upwards into the outflow tract.*

narrowed subpulmonary outflow tract

septal attachment

infundibular septum

ventriculo-infundibular fold

anterior limb & body of septomarginal trabecula

posterior limb & medial papillary muscle

overriding aortic valve

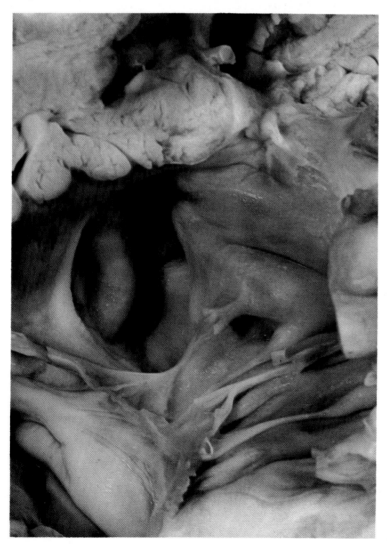

infundibular septum

overriding aortic valve

ventriculo-infundibular fold

remnant of inter-ventricular membranous septum

septomarginal trabecula

conduction tissue axis

atrio-ventricular node

Fig. 6.50 *Boundaries of perimembranous ventricular septal defect in tetralogy of Fallot, in surgical orientation. The septal leaflet of the tricuspid valve has been removed and the conduction tissue axis superimposed.*

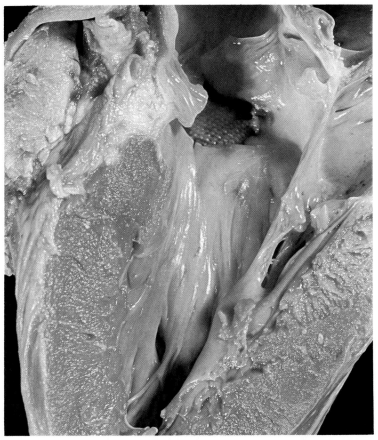

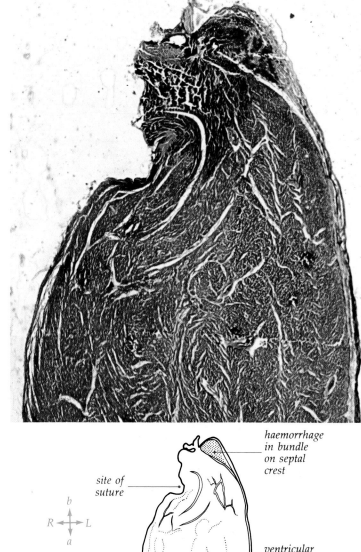

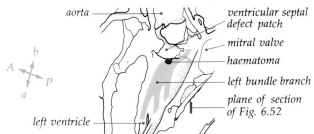

aorta — ventricular septal defect patch

— mitral valve

— haematoma

— left bundle branch

— plane of section of Fig. 6.52

left ventricle —

A ← → P, b/a

site of suture —

haemorrhage in bundle on septal crest

ventricular septum

R ← → L, b/a

Fig. 6.51 *Left ventricular aspect of heart with tetralogy of Fallot which was repaired by suturing directly to the septal crest.*

Fig. 6.52 *Histological section from heart in Fig. 6.51 shows interruption of the conduction axis, which was unusually situated directly astride the septum, by one of the sutures. Trichrome stain.*

form of a waist-like narrowing of the pulmonary trunk just distal to the valve, though it may occur anywhere at one or more locations within the pulmonary arterial tree. Narrowing has also been reported within collateral vessels supplying the lung directly from the aorta in cases of pulmonary atresia and ventricular septal defect (*Haworth & Macartney, 1980*). Very rarely, membrane-like obstructions may be found, but the usual lesion is more akin to a segmental tubular hypoplasia. These lesions, if anatomically accessible, are amenable to simple patch grafting.

One form of right ventricular outflow tract obstruction is so clearly demarcated that it constitutes an entity in its own right, namely tetralogy of Fallot. Its anatomical hallmark is anterosuperior deviation of the septal insertion of the infundibular septum (*Becker, Connor & Anderson, 1975*). In the normal heart (Fig. 6.48), this structure is firmly anchored to the trabecular septum between the limbs of the septomarginal trabecula and is fused with the ventriculo-

infundibular fold (see Figs. 2.27 & 2.28). It is the alignment of these three structures (infundibular septum, ventriculo-infundibular fold and septomarginal trabecula) which produces the normal supraventricular crest in continuity with the so-called 'septal band'.

In tetralogy of Fallot, the infundibular septal insertion into the trabecular septum occurs along or superior to the anterior limb of the septomarginal trabecula. In a single stroke this deviation divorces the infundibular septum from the ventriculo-infundibular fold, narrows the sub-pulmonary outflow tract, opens up a ventricular septal defect and results in overriding of the aortic valve (Fig. 6.49).

The ventricular defect is consequently a malalignment outlet defect, either perimembranous or with a muscular posteroinferior rim (*Anderson et al., 1981*), according to the nature of its posteroinferior angle. These features have the same implications for conduction tissue disposition as they do in isolated ventricular septal defects (see Chapter 6,

ii). When the defect is perimembranous, the posteroinferior margin is the area of aortic-mitral-tricuspid valve continuity and the atrioventricular conduction axis penetrates beneath the atrioventricular membranous component of this fibrous area (Fig. 6.50). Usually, in tetralogy the non-branching bundle and the branching bundle are carried down the left ventricular side of the septum some distance from the septal crest. In a minority of cases the bundle can branch directly astride the septum (*Titus, Daugherty & Edwards, 1963; Anderson et al., 1977*) and can then be traumatized by sutures placed directly onto the septal crest (Figs. 6.51 & 6.52).

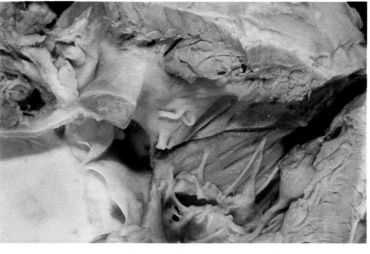

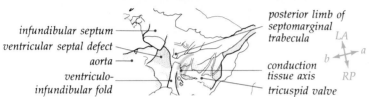

infundibular septum
ventricular septal defect
aorta
ventriculo-
infundibular fold

posterior limb of
septomarginal
trabecula

conduction
tissue axis

tricuspid valve

LA
b — a
RP

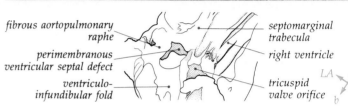

fibrous aortopulmonary
raphe

perimembranous
ventricular septal defect

ventriculo-
infundibular fold

septomarginal
trabecula

right ventricle

tricuspid
valve orifice

LA
a
RP
b

Fig. 6.53 *Defect in tetralogy of Fallot with a muscular posteroinferior rim, in surgical orientation.*

Fig. 6.54 *Opened outflow tracts showing a doubly-committed subarterial defect which extends to become perimembranous, in surgical orientation.*

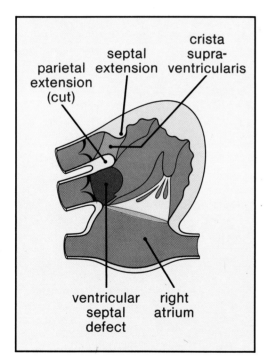

crista
supra-
ventricularis

septal
extension

parietal
extension
(cut)

ventricular
septal
defect

right
atrium

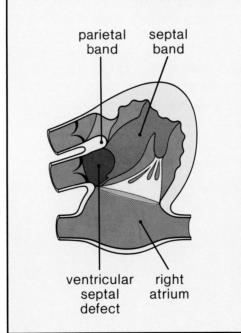

parietal
band

septal
band

ventricular
septal
defect

right
atrium

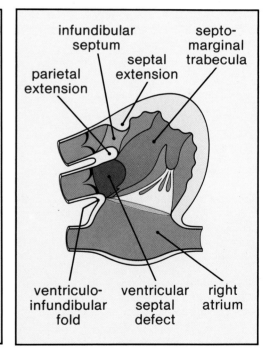

infundibular
septum

septo-
marginal
trabecula

septal
extension

parietal
extension

ventriculo-
infundibular
fold

ventricular
septal
defect

right
atrium

Fig. 6.55 *Nomenclature for the muscle bundles of the outflow tract in tetralogy used by Kjellberg and his colleagues.*

Fig. 6.56 *Nomenclature suggested by Van Praagh for the outflow tract muscle bundles in tetralogy.*

Fig. 6.57 *Our proposed nomenclature, which avoids potential confusion concerning the nature of the 'septal' or 'parietal' bands.*

In about one-fifth of cases of tetralogy, the defect is not perimembranous. In these hearts, the posterior limb of the septomarginal trabecula fuses with the ventriculoinfundibular fold superior to an intact interventricular membranous septum, thus protecting the atrioventricular conduction tissues (Fig. 6.53). Superficial sutures can be placed along the entire margin of the right ventricular aspect of the defect without fear of traumatizing the conduction tissues. In rare cases, more frequently encountered in the Far East or South America (*Ando, 1974; Neirotti et al.,*

1978), the infundibular septum is absent and the defect becomes doubly-committed and subarterial (Fig. 6.54). Although strictly speaking these are questionable examples of tetralogy, the significant feature concerning the conduction tissue is the posteroinferior margin. Again, the inferior border of the defect may be either muscular or perimembranous.

While it is clearly important to close securely the ventricular septal defect in tetralogy, probably the most important feature for a successful surgical outcome

is relief of the pulmonary outflow obstruction. One of the major determinants of this success is the size of the pulmonary trunk. Tables are now available for preoperative evaluation to select those hearts which can be successfully corrected (*Blackstone et al., 1979; Kirklin et al., 1979*). An understanding of the precise anatomy of the subpulmonary outflow tract is vital if the surgeon is to plan accurately a reproducible operation for successful relief of the obstruction.

A clear understanding of the various accounts of the surgery required in this

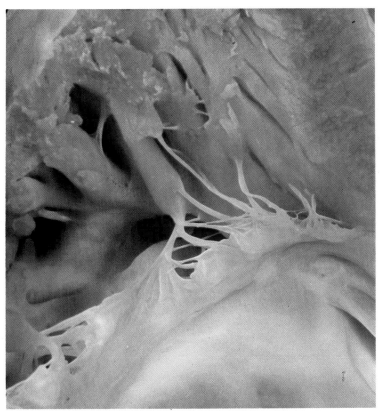

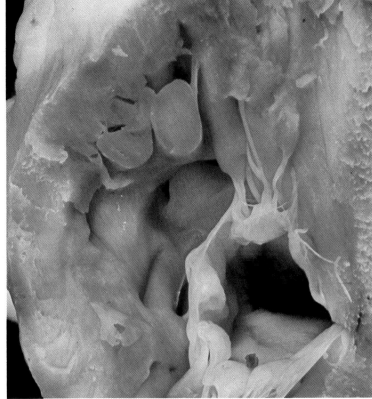

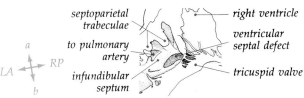

septoparietal trabeculae

right ventricle

to pulmonary artery

ventricular septal defect

infundibular septum

tricuspid valve

a

LA — *RP*

b

Fig. 6.58 *Obstructed subpulmonary outflow tract in tetralogy, as seen from the right ventricular apex.*

septoparietal trabeculae

ventricular septal defect & aortic valve

to pulmonary trunk

ventriculoinfundibular fold

infundibular septum

tricuspid valve

a

LA — *RP*

b

Fig. 6.59 *Further dissection showing the trabeculae which produce parietal obstruction.*

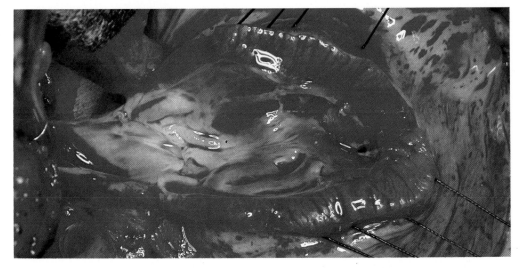

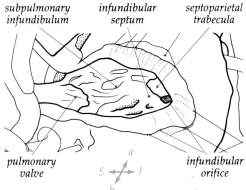

subpulmonary infundibulum

infundibular septum

septoparietal trabecula

pulmonary valve

infundibular orifice

a

S — *I*

b

Fig. 6.60 *Operative view of subpulmonary obstruction in tetralogy, seen through a transvalvular incision.*

area has been hampered by the rather indiscriminate use of the term 'crista'. Some angiocardiographers use the term 'septal band' for the anterior part of the subpulmonary obstruction. This is a completely different structure from the 'septal band' described by Van Praagh (1968). The term 'crista' was used by Kjellberg and his colleagues (1959) in describing the insertion of the infundibular septum into the trabecular septum where the body of the septum itself was considered the 'crista' (Fig. 6.55). In contrast, Van Praagh labelled the entire infundibular septum (the 'crista' of Kjellberg) as the 'parietal band', reserving the term 'septal band' for the structure we now call the septomarginal trabecula (Fig. 6.56).

The potential confusion is avoided by using descriptive terms which define the situation more accurately (Fig. 6.57). From the surgical point of view, the angiocardiographic interpretation of Kjellberg et al. (1959) is probably misleadingly simplistic. It is a frequent assumption that the two insertions of the infundibular septum meet in the superior free wall of the right ventricle, forming a 'lasso' around the orifice of the subpulmonary outflow tract and producing a constrictive muscular orifice. Examination of hearts shows that this is probably not so (Fig. 6.58). Certainly a constrictive muscular annulus is formed, but its parietal segment is produced by hypertrophy of free-standing septoparietal trabeculations (Fig. 6.59). This is important to the surgeon when deciding which muscle to resect in order to widen the subpulmonary outflow tract (Fig. 6.60).

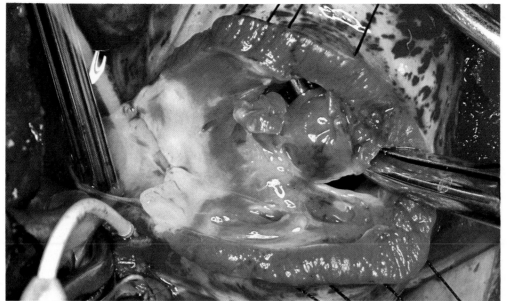

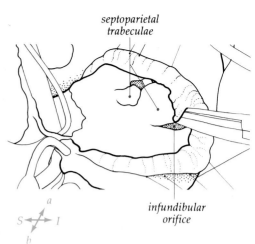

Fig. 6.61 *Operative view of septoparietal trabeculae, which can be liberated and removed.*

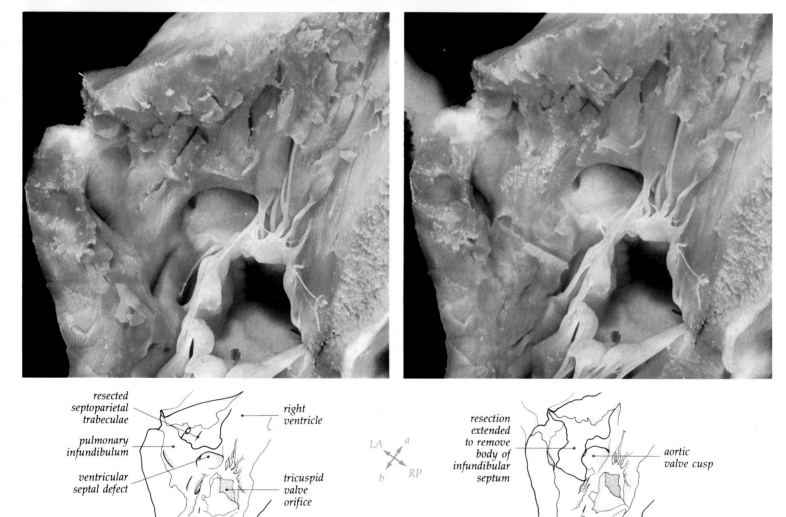

Fig. 6.62 *Appearance of the heart in Fig. 6.59 after removal of the septoparietal trabeculae, seen in a more or less surgical orientation.*

Fig. 6.63 *Excision of the body of the outlet septum brings the surgeon perilously close to the aortic valve, orientated as in Fig. 6.62.*

The major limiting structure is always the hypertrophied septal insertion of the infundibular septum, which can be dissected without fear of damaging vital structures. At the same time, any free-standing septoparietal trabeculations should certainly be identified and removed since they, too, never contain vital structures (Figs. 6.61 & 6.62). The body of the infundibular septum ('crista')

usually contributes to obstruction and ideally should be resected. However, excessive resection of this structure may lead to damage to the aortic valve leaflets arising from its left ventricular aspect (Fig. 6.63).

It is also usual to resect the parietal insertion of the infundibular septum (Fig. 6.64). This fuses with the ventriculo-infundibular fold, which is the inner

curvature of the heart; care must be taken not to perforate through to the transverse sinus (*McFadden, Culpepper & Ochsner, 1982*). It is very unusual for the septomarginal trabecula itself (the 'septal band') to contribute to the infundibular obstruction and, therefore, it is usually unnecessary to resect its limbs. Nonetheless, its body and the moderator band may be hypertrophied, particularly

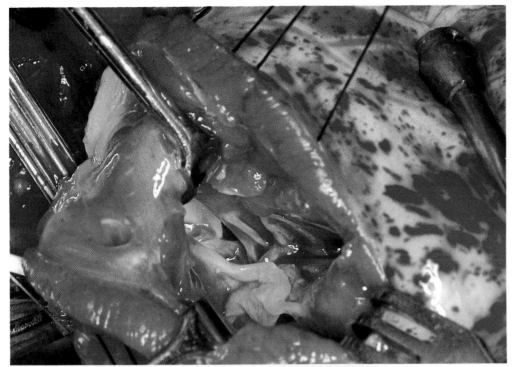

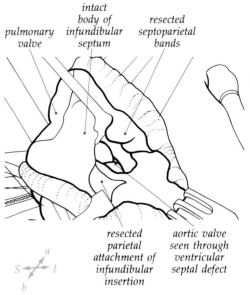

Fig. 6.64 *Operative view after completion of resection of parietal insertion of the outlet (infundibular) septum.*

intact
body of
infundibular
septum

pulmonary
valve

resected
septoparietal
bands

resected
parietal
attachment of
infundibular
insertion

aortic valve
seen through
ventricular
septal defect

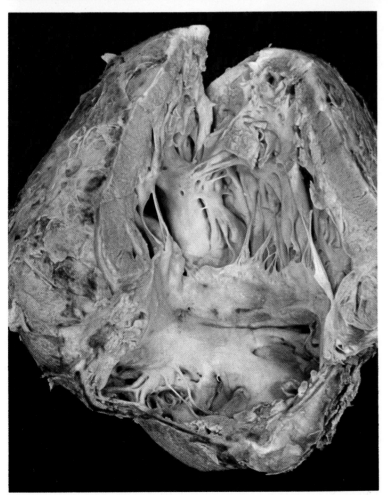

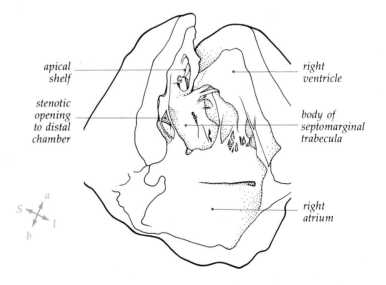

apical
shelf

right
ventricle

stenotic
opening
to distal
chamber

body of
septomarginal
trabecula

right
atrium

Fig. 6.65 *Opened right atrioventricular junction, in approximately surgical orientation, showing severe hypertrophy of the body of the septomarginal trabecula and moderator band, producing 'two-chambered right ventricle'.*

when the latter structure has a high take-off. Severe hypertrophy produces a two-chambered right ventricle and the intervening 'septum' may require resection (Fig. 6.65). The anterior papillary muscle of the tricuspid valve often arises from the inlet aspect of the obstructing shelf; care must be taken not to damage this muscle in resection.

The final variable in tetralogy of Fallot is the degree of aortic override. This varies from the aorta being connected mostly to the left ventricle (concordant ventriculo-arterial connexion) to its being connected mostly to the right ventricle (double outlet connexion). The degree of override should not markedly affect the surgical procedure although, with greater commit-ment of the aorta to the right ventricle, the placement of the ventricular septal patch becomes more important. The 'internal conduit' from the left ventricle to the aorta

may further complicate relief of the right ventricular outflow obstruction.

Although the primary obstruction in tetralogy is at the infundibular level, the pulmonary valve is frequently stenotic and this must be relieved during operative repair. The sequelae of postoperative pulmonary regurgitation are not yet clearly established, but they are certainly less troublesome than those of residual pulmonary stenosis.

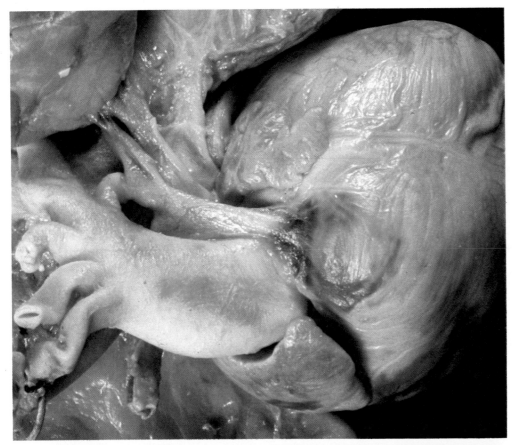

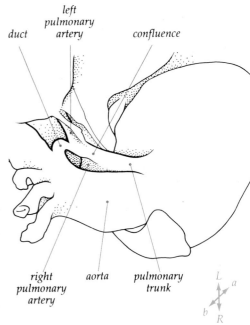

Fig. 6.66 *Duct supplying pulmonary arteries in pulmonary atresia with ventricular septal defect, in surgical orientation.*

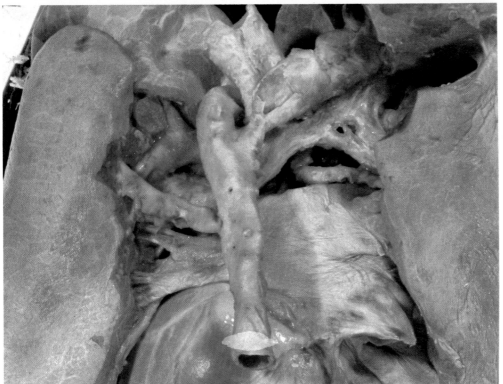

Fig. 6.67 *Posterior aspect of anatomically orientated descending aorta in pulmonary atresia with ventricular septal defect showing two major aortopulmonary collateral arteries.*

The most common type of pulmonary atresia with ventricular septal defect is, in essence, tetralogy of Fallot with infundibular pulmonary atresia and is described as such by some authorities (*Alfieri et al., 1978*). The ventricular anatomy includes deviation of the infundibular septum sufficient to block completely the subpulmonary infundibulum. The anatomy of the ventricular septal defect can vary as in tetralogy, but the intracardiac anatomy is of relatively minor surgical significance. The feature

which dominates the surgical options is the morphology of the pulmonary arteries. Although exceedingly rarely the pulmonary arteries may be supplied through a persistent fifth arch (*Macartney, Scott & Deverall, 1974*) or an aortopulmonary window, in essence the lungs are supplied either through a duct or through major aortopulmonary collateral arteries. Rarely, a duct and collateral arteries can supply the same lung. When a duct is present and the pulmonary arteries are confluent (Fig. 6.66), the arteries supply the lung

parenchyma and are variably developed. The degree of hypoplasia determines whether total correction is feasible.

When the right and left pulmonary arteries are not confluent or when major aortopulmonary collateral arteries are present, the situation is more complex. Non-confluent pulmonary arteries can be supplied independently by a bilateral duct, or one lung can be supplied by a duct and the other through collateral arteries. It is more usual for collateral arteries (Fig. 6.67) to supply both lungs

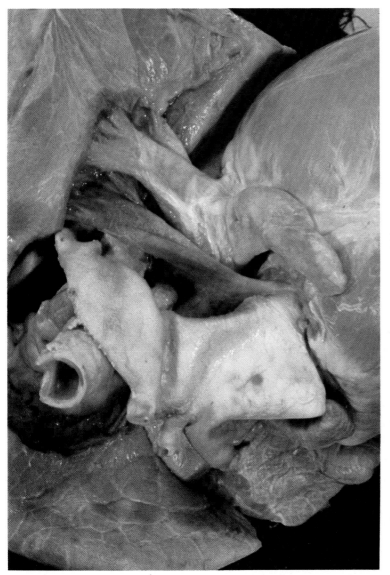

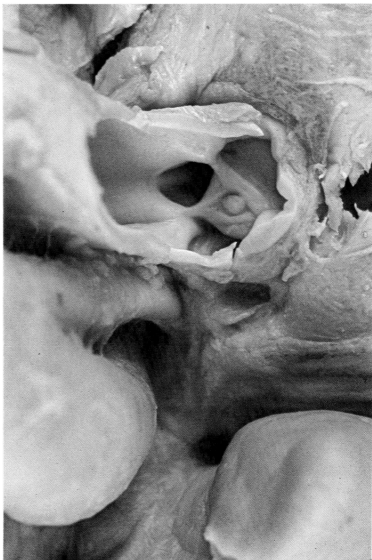

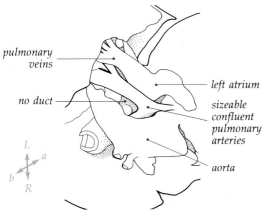

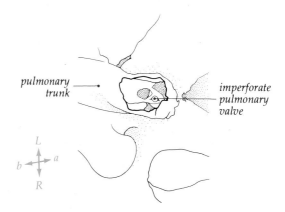

Fig. 6.68 *Base of heart seen in Fig. 6.67 showing large confluent pulmonary arteries but without duct. The arteries are fed by a large right-sided collateral artery (not visible here).*

Fig. 6.69 *Imperforate pulmonary valve in pulmonary atresia with intact septum, in surgical orientation.*

with no duct being present.

Well developed confluent pulmonary arteries may coexist with collateral arteries (Fig. 6.68). The important point to establish is how much of the lung parenchyma is connected to the pulmonary arteries and how much is supplied directly by collateral arteries. It is known that collateral arteries can anastomose with the pulmonary arteries at the hilum or extend into the parenchyma to supply lobar or segmental

arteries directly. Also, intersegmental anastomoses occur. The object of preoperative evaluation should therefore be to establish precisely how much of each lung is supplied by the central pulmonary arteries (*Haworth & Macartney, 1980*), since this is the ultimate determinant of the success of the attempted total correction.

In contrast to pulmonary atresia with ventricular septal defect where initial survival is good and the results of surgery

are continually improving, pulmonary atresia with intact septum has a grave prognosis. The results of attempted corrective surgery are uniformly poor (*Dobell & Grignon, 1977; Moulton et al., 1979*). The anatomy of the lesion itself accounts for the dismal outcome (*Freedom, Dische & Rowe, 1978; Zuberbuhler & Anderson, 1979*).

The atresia can be due either to an imperforate pulmonary valve membrane (Fig. 6.69) or to infundibular atresia. In

6.29

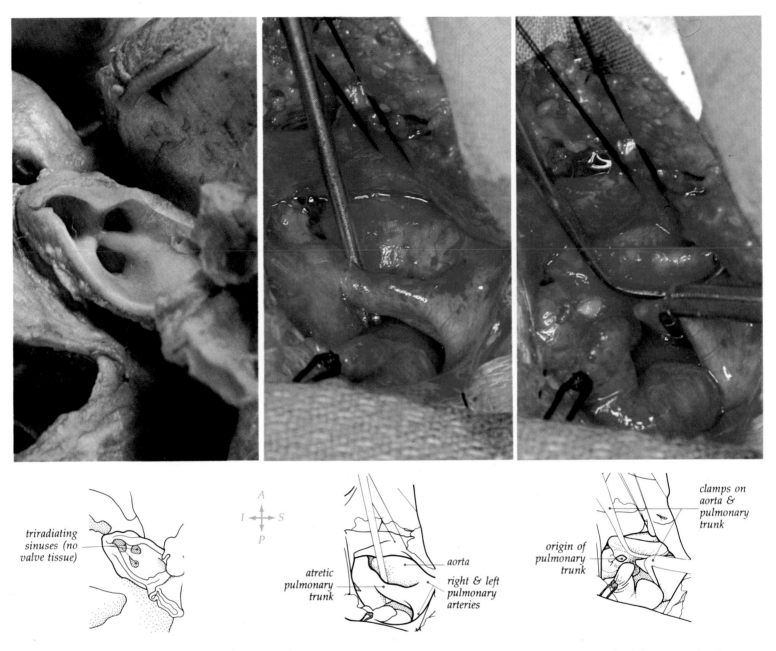

Fig. 6.70 *(Left) atretic pulmonary trunk in surgical orientation shows triradiating ridges of sinuses of Valsalva but no valve; (middle) pulmonary trunk leading back to ventricular surface of a small right ventricle, seen through a left thoracotomy; (right) transected pulmonary trunk shows no valve tissue or blood flow from its opened origin.*

the latter, the pulmonary trunk is blind-ending with no vestiges of pulmonary valve tissue (Fig. 6.70). The outlet and trabecular parts of the right ventricle are more or less completely obliterated by gross hypertrophy of the ventricular wall and the cavity is effectively represented only by the hypoplastic inlet portion (Fig. 6.71). This cavity is unlikely ever to perform a useful function and should probably be disregarded when deciding surgical treatment (*de Leval et al., 1982*). When there is an imperforate pulmonary valve, a spectrum of cavity size is seen. In some hearts, hypertrophy of the right ventricular myocardium obliterates the trabecular part of the cavity and it is questionable if these ventricles will ever grow and become useful (*Bull et al., 1982*). In the most favourable situation, the cavity is less hypoplastic and has well developed inlet, trabecular and outlet components (Fig. 6.72). These cases are most amenable to total operative correction.

Whatever the intracardiac anatomy, it is rarely that one finds the thread-like pulmonary arteries seen so frequently with pulmonary atresia with ventricular septal defect. Furthermore, the pulmonary blood flow is almost always duct-dependent. With prostaglandin therapy now available to improve ductal flow, the pulmonary arteries are almost always of sufficient size to permit construction of a systemic-pulmonary shunt. Other options, such as the need for pulmonary valvotomy, should be decided after assessment of the precise anatomy of the individual case (*de Leval et al., 1982*).

Pulmonary valvular insufficiency may be congenital or acquired, the latter usually secondary to surgical intervention or pulmonary hypertension. Congenital pulmonary valvular insufficiency may be associated with marked deformity of the valve tissue, as in valvular dysplasia, or with absence of the valve tissue altogether. Rudimentary cusps may be seen with an intact ventricular septum (*Smith, DuShane & Edwards, 1959*) or in combination with ventricular septal defect (Fig. 6.73). Absence of the pulmonary valve leaflets is also found in combination with tetralogy of Fallot (*Macartney & Miller, 1970*).

While gross pulmonary valvular insufficiency may be tolerated by the right heart relatively well, it can result in marked enlargement of the pulmonary trunk and arteries. Indeed, compromise of the tracheobronchial tree by these grossly enlarged vessels results in most patients presenting with symptoms of respiratory distress. Because only a limited number of cases have come to surgical correction, the efficacy of valve replacement with or without arterial plication has not been proved (*Goor & Lillehei, 1975*). Fortunately this is a rare condition.

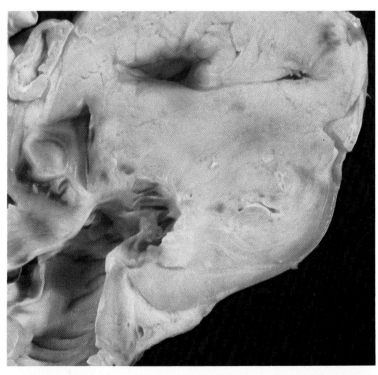

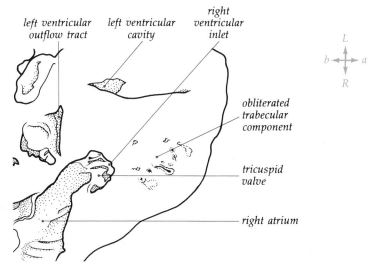

left ventricular outflow tract left ventricular cavity right ventricular inlet

obliterated trabecular component

tricuspid valve

right atrium

Fig. 6.71 *Long-axis section at right angles to the septum in approximate surgical orientation showing overgrowth and obliteration of right ventricular trabecular component in pulmonary atresia with intact ventricular septum.*

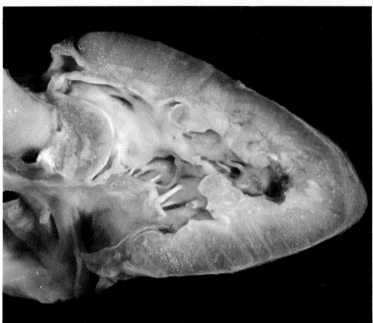

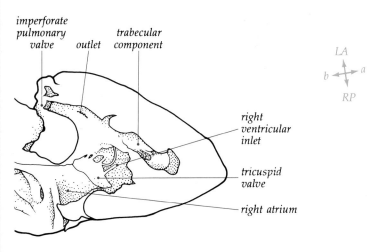

imperforate pulmonary valve outlet trabecular component

right ventricular inlet

tricuspid valve

right atrium

Fig. 6.72 *Pulmonary atresia with intact septum in which the cavity has all of its (albeit somewhat hypoplastic) components present.*

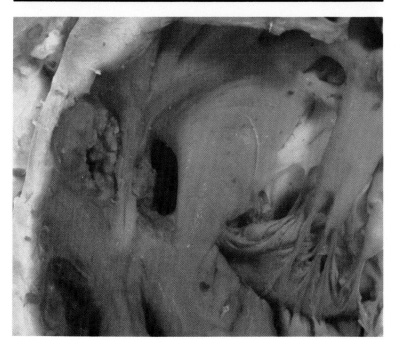

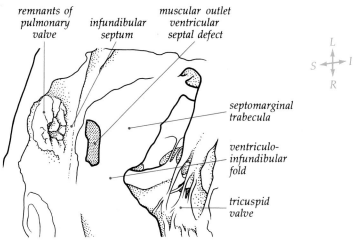

remnants of pulmonary valve infundibular septum muscular outlet ventricular septal defect

septomarginal trabecula

ventriculo-infundibular fold

tricuspid valve

Fig. 6.73 *Right ventricular outflow tract in surgical orientation showing absent pulmonary valve and muscular outlet ventricular septal defect.*

Alfieri, O., Blackstone, E.H., Kirklin, J.W., Pacifico, A.D. & Bargeron, L.M. Jr. (1978) Surgical treatment of tetralogy of Fallot with pulmonary atresia. *Journal of Thoracic and Cardiovascular Surgery*, **76**, 321–335.

Anderson, R.H., Allwork, S.P., Ho, S.Y., Lenox, C.C. & Zuberbuhler, J.R. (1981) Surgical anatomy of tetralogy of Fallot. *Journal of Thoracic and Cardiovascular Surgery*, **81**, 887–896.

Anderson, R.H., Lenox, C.C. & Zuberbuhler, J.R. (1983) Mechanisms of closure of perimembranous ventricular septal defects. *American Journal of Cardiology*, **52**, 341–345.

Anderson, R.H., Monro, J.L., Ho, S.Y., Smith, A. & Deverall, P.B. (1977) Les voies de conduction auriculo-ventriculaires dans le tetralogie de Fallot. *Coeur*, **8**, 793–807.

Ando, M. (1974) Subpulmonary ventricular septal defect with pulmonary stenosis. Letter to Editor. *Circulation*, **50**, 412.

Becker, A.E. (1983) Valve pathology in the paediatric age group. In *Paediatric Cardiology*, pp 345–360. Edited by R.H. Anderson, F.J. Macartney, E.A. Shinebourne & M.J. Tynan. Edinburgh: Churchill Livingstone.

Becker, A.E. & Anderson, R.H. (1981) *Pathology of Congenital Heart Disease*, pp 137–163. London: Butterworths.

Becker, A.E. & Anderson, R.H. (1982) Atrioventricular septal defects. What's in a name? *Journal of Thoracic and Cardiovascular Surgery*, **83**, 461–469.

Becker, A.E., Connor, M. & Anderson, R.H. (1975) Tetralogy of Fallot: a morphometric and geometric study. *American Journal of Cardiology*, **35**, 402–412.

Becu, L.M., Fontana, R.S., DuShane, J.W., Kirklin, J.W., Burchell, H.B. & Edwards, J.E. (1956) Anatomic and pathologic studies in ventricular septal defect. *Circulation*, **14**, 349–364.

Bharati, S. & Lev, M. (1973) The spectrum of common atrioventricular orifice (canal). *American Heart Journal*, **86**, 553–561.

Bharati, S., Lev, M., McAllister, H.A. Jr. & Kirklin, J.W. (1980) Surgical anatomy of the atrioventricular valve in the intermediate type of common atrioventricular orifice. *Journal of Thoracic and Cardiovascular Surgery*, **79**, 884–889.

Blackstone, E.H., Kirklin, J.W., Bertranou, E.G., Labrosse, C.J., Soto, B. & Bargeron, L.M. Jr. (1979) Preoperative prediction from cineangiograms of post-repair right ventricular pressure in tetralogy of Fallot. *Journal of Thoracic and Cardiovascular Surgery*, **78**, 542–552.

Brandt, P.W.T., Clarkson, P.M., Neutze, J.M. & Barratt-Boyes, B.G. (1972) Left ventricular cineangiography in endocardial cushion defect (persistent common atrioventricular canal). *Australasian Radiology*, **16**, 367–376.

Bull, C., de Leval, M.R., Mercanti, C., Macartney, F.J. & Anderson, R.H. (1982) Pulmonary atresia and intact ventricular septum: a revised classification. *Circulation*, **66**, 266–271.

de Leval, M.R., Bull, C., Stark, J., Anderson, R.H., Taylor, J.F.N. & Macartney, F.J. (1982) Pulmonary atresia and intact ventricular septum: surgical management based on a revised classification. *Circulation*, **66**, 272–280.

Dobell, A.R.C. & Grignon, A. (1977) Early and late results in pulmonary atresia. *Annals of Thoracic Surgery*, **24**, 264–274.

Doty, D.B., Polansky, D.B. & Jenson, C.B. (1977) Supravalvular aortic stenosis. Repair by extended aortoplasty. *Journal of Thoracic and Cardiovascular Surgery*, **74**, 362–371.

Edwards, J.E. (1965) Pathology of left ventricular outflow obstruction. *Circulation*, **31**, 586–599.

Frantz, P.J., Murray, G.F. & Wilcox, B.R. (1980) Surgical management of left ventricular-aortic discontinuity complicating bacterial endocarditis. *Annals of Thoracic Surgery*, **29**, 1–7.

Freedom, R.M., Dische, M.R. & Rowe, R.D. (1978) The tricuspid valve in pulmonary atresia with intact ventricular septum. A morphological study of 60 cases. *Archives of Pathology and Laboratory Medicine*, **102**, 28–31.

Gilbert, J.W., Morrow, A.G. & Talbert, J.W. (1963) The surgical significance of hypertrophic infundibular obstruction accompanying valvar pulmonary stenosis. *Journal of Thoracic and Cardiovascular Surgery*, **46**, 457–467.

Goor, D.A. & Lillehei, C.W. (1975) Pulmonary valvular insufficiency. In *Congenital Malformations of the Heart*, pp 336–339. New York: Grune and Stratton.

Haworth, S.G. & Macartney, F.J. (1980) Growth and development of pulmonary circulation in pulmonary atresia with ventricular septal defect and major aortopulmonary collateral arteries. *British Heart Journal*, **44**, 14–24.

Kirklin, J.W., Blackstone, E.H., Pacifico, A.D., Brown, R.N. & Bargeron, L.M. Jr. (1979) Routine primary repair vs two-stage repair of tetralogy of Fallot. *Circulation*, **60**, 373–385.

Kjellberg, S.R., Mannheimer, E., Rudhe, U. & Jonsson, B. (1959) *Diagnosis of Congenital Heart Disease, 2nd edition*. Chicago: Year Book Medical Publishers.

Layman, T.E. & Edwards, J.E. (1967) Anomalous mitral arcade: A type of congenital mitral insufficiency. *Circulation*, **35**, 389–395.

Macartney, F.J. & Miller, G.A.H. (1970) Congenital absence of the pulmonary valve. *British Heart Journal*, **32**, 483–490.

Macartney, F.J., Scott, O. & Deverall, P.B. (1974) Haemodynamic and anatomical characteristics of pulmonary blood supply in pulmonary atresia with ventricular septal defect – including a case of persistent fifth aortic arch. *British Heart Journal*, **36**, 1049–1060.

McFadden, P.M., Culpepper, W.S. & Ochsner, J.L. (1982) Iatrogenic right ventricular failure in tetralogy of Fallot repairs: reappraisal of a distressing problem. *Annals of Thoracic Surgery*, **33**, 400–402.

McGoon, D.C., Danielson, G.K., Wallace, R.B. & Puga, F.J. (1981) Surgical implications of straddling atrioventricular valves. In *Paediatric Cardiology Volume 3*, pp 431–448. Edited by A. E. Becker, G. Losekoot, C. Marcelletti & R.H. Anderson. Edinburgh: Churchill Livingstone.

McKay, R. & Ross D.N. (1982) Technique for the relief of discrete subaortic stenosis. *Journal of Thoracic and Cardiovascular Surgery*, **84**, 917–920.

Milo, S., Ho, S.Y., Wilkinson, J.L. & Anderson, R.H. (1980) The surgical anatomy and atrioventricular conduction tissues of hearts with isolated ventricular septal defects. *Journal of Thoracic and Cardiovascular Surgery*, **79**, 244–255.

Morrow, A.G., Waldhausen, J.A., Peters, R.L., Bloodwell, R.D. & Braunwald, E. (1959) Supravalvular aortic stenosis. *Circulation*, **20**, 1003–1010.

Moulaert, A.J. & Oppenheimer-Dekker, A. (1976) Anterolateral muscle bundle of the left ventricle, bulboventricular flange and subaortic stenosis. *American Journal of Cardiology*, **37**, 78–81.

Moulton, A.L., Bowman, F.O., Edie, R.N., Hayes, C.J., Ellis, K., Gersony, W.M. & Malm, J. (1979) Pulmonary atresia with intact ventricular septum. Sixteen-year experience. *Journal of Thoracic and Cardiovascular Surgery*, **78**, 527–536.

Neirotti, R., Galindez, E., Kreutzer, G., Coronel, A.R., Pedrini, M. & Becu, L. (1978) Tetralogy of Fallot with sub-pulmonary ventricular septal defect. *Annals of Thoracic Surgery*, **25**, 51–56.

Pacifico, A.D., Soto, B. & Bargeron, L.M. Jr. (1979) Surgical treatment of straddling tricuspid valves. *Circulation*, **60**, 655–664.

Piccoli, G.P., Ho, S.Y., Wilkinson, J.L., Macartney, F.J., Gerlis, L.M. & Anderson, R.H. (1982) Left-sided obstructive lesions in atrioventricular septal defects. *Journal of Thoracic and Cardiovascular Surgery*, **83**, 453–460.

Piccoli, G.P., Wilkinson, J.L., Macartney, F.J., Gerlis, L.M. & Anderson, R.H. (1979) Morphology and classification of complete atrioventricular defects. *British Heart Journal*, **42**, 633–639.

Pillai, R., Ho, S.Y., Anderson, R.H., Shinebourne, E.A. & Lincoln, C. (1984) Malalignment of the interventricular septum with atrioventricular septal defect: its implications concerning conduction tissue disposition. *Journal of Thoracic and Cardiovascular Surgery*, **32**, 1–3.

Quaegebeur, J., Kirklin, J.W., Pacifico, A.D. & Bargeron, L.M. Jr. (1979) Surgical experience with unroofed coronary sinus. *Annals of Thoracic Surgery*, **27**, 418–425.

Rastelli, G.C., Kirklin, J.W. & Titus, J.L. (1966) Anatomic observations on complete form of persistent common atrioventricular canal with special reference to atrioventricular valves. *Mayo Clinic Proceedings*, **41**, 296–308.

Rosenquist, G.C. (1974) Overriding right atrioventricular valve in association with mitral atresia. *American Heart Journal*, **87**, 26–32.

Ruckman, R.N. & Van Praagh, R. (1978) Anatomic types of congenital mitral stenosis: report of 49 cases with consideration of diagnosis and surgical implications. *American Journal of Cardiology*, **42**, 592–601.

Ruschaupt, D.G., Bharati, S. & Lev, M. (1976) Mitral valve malformation of Ebstein type in absence of corrected transposition. *American Journal of Cardiology*, **38**, 109–112.

Shone, J., Sellers, R., Anderson, R.C., Adams, P., Lillehei, C.W. & Edwards, J.E. (1963) The developmental complex of parachute mitral valve. *American Journal of Cardiology*, **11**, 714–725.

Smith, R.D., DuShane, J.W. & Edwards J.E. (1959) Congenital insufficiency of the pulmonary valve: including a case of fetal cardiac failure. *Circulation*, **20**, 554–560

Soto, B., Becker, A.E., Moulaert, A.J., Lie, J.T. & Anderson, R.H. (1980) Classification of ventricular septal defects. *British Heart Journal*, **43**, 332–343.

Titus, J.L., Daugherty, G.W. & Edwards, J.E. (1963) Anatomy of the atrioventricular conduction system in ventricular septal defect. *Circulation*, **28**, 72–81

Van Mierop, L.H.S. (1970) Pathology and pathogenesis of the common cardiac malformations. In *Cardiovascular Clinics Volume 2.1*, pp 27–60. Edited by A.N. Brest & D. Downing. Philadelphia: F.A. Davis Company.

Van Praagh, R. (1968) What is the Taussig-Bing malformation? *Circulation*, **38**, 445–449.

Van Praagh, R & McNamara, J.J. (1968) Anatomic types of ventricular septal defects with aortic insufficiency. Diagnostic and surgical considerations. *American Heart Journal*, **73**, 604–619

Vollebergh, F.E.M.G. & Becker, A.E. (1977) Minor congenital variations of cusp size in tricuspid aortic valves. Possible link with isolated aortic stenosis. *British Heart Journal*, **39**, 1006–1011.

Wakai, C.S. & Edwards, J.E. (1956) Developmental and pathologic considerations in persistent common atrioventricular canal. *Mayo Clinic Proceedings*, **31**, 487–500.

Zuberbuhler, J.R. & Anderson, R.H. (1979) Morphological variations in pulmonary atresia with intact ventricular septum. *British Heart Journal*, **41**, 281–288.

7 Lesions in Abnormally Connected Hearts

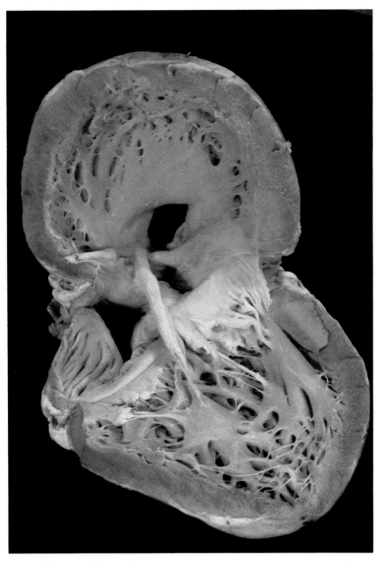

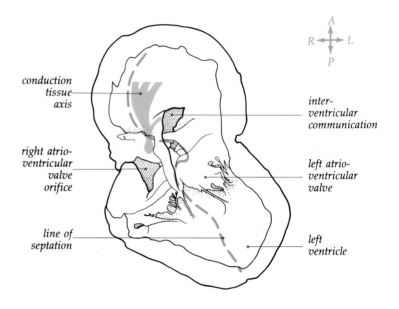

conduction tissue axis

inter-ventricular communication

right atrio-ventricular valve orifice

left atrio-ventricular valve

line of septation

left ventricle

Fig. 7.1 *Dominant left ventricle with double inlet opened in 'fishmouth' fashion. The course of the conduction tissue axis, together with the position of a path for complete septation, are superimposed (see also Fig. 7.4).*

i. Double inlet ventricle

As the name suggests, this is the atrioventricular connexion in which both atria are connected to the same ventricle. Hearts with straddling valves can also have a double inlet connexion when all of one atrium and the greater part of the other are connected to the same ventricle. Double inlet ventricle can exist with any atrial arrangement, with the connexions effected by two atrioventricular valves or a common valve, with variable ventricular morphology and with any ventriculo-arterial connexion (*Anderson et al., 1979; Girod et al., 1984*). All of these influence the success of attempted surgical repair, but the most significant differentiating feature is ventricular morphology. On this basis three subsets can be distinguished: those with the atria connected to a left ventricle; those with the atria connected to a right ventricle; and those with the atria connected to a morphologically indeterminate ventricle. Operations have been performed most frequently on hearts with a dominant left ventricle ('single ventricle with outlet chamber') and this is the variant we will discuss.

It is important to note that with double inlet left ventricle (Fig. 7.1) there is almost invariably an anterosuperior rudimentary right ventricle with a trabecular septum

between the ventricles that does not extend to the crux. The features determining the potential success of attempted correction are the state of the atrioventricular valves, the position of the rudimentary ventricle, the site of the interventricular communication relative to the atrioventricular valves, the ventriculo-arterial connexion, the state of the ventricular outflow tracts and the disposition of the atrioventricular conduction tissues. The options for surgical correction are either a modified Fontan procedure (*Gale et al., 1979*) or a septation procedure (*Danielson et al., 1978; McKay et al., 1982*). The former is available for the greater majority of hearts with double inlet left ventricle since the only anatomical requisites are to isolate the systemic venous atrium and connect it to the pulmonary arterial supply. Ideally, in those with concordant ventriculoarterial connexions ('Holmes hearts') the rudimentary right ventricle (Fig. 7.2) should be incorporated into the new pulmonary circulation as is done in hearts with classical tricuspid atresia. In hearts without ventriculoarterial concordance, the right atrioventricular valve should be closed (or the right component of a common valve excluded from the systemic venous atrium) and the right

atrium connected directly to the pulmonary trunk. Often, depending on the relationship of the great arteries, this can be achieved by direct anastomosis of the right atrial appendage to the pulmonary trunk (*Doty, Marvin & Lauer, 1981*). When closing the right atrio-ventricular valve the site of the anomalously connecting atrioventricular node is important to the surgeon (Fig. 7.3). Although the anatomy in most cases permits a modified Fontan procedure (*Girod et al., 1984*), many hearts will be ruled out because they do not fulfil the haemodynamic criteria (*Fontan et al., 1978*).

The presence of many associated lesions prevents septation in most cases because experience has shown that, for a reasonable chance of success, two 'normal' atrioventricular valves are a vital prerequisite. Many cases have ventriculo-arterial discordance (transposition) and only those with anterior or left-sided rudimentary right ventricles are suitable for septation. An unrestrictive inter-ventricular communication is also needed (*Stefanelli et al., 1984*). The septation patch can then be placed between the atrio-ventricular valves to connect the right valve to the subpulmonary outflow tract and the left valve to the interventricular

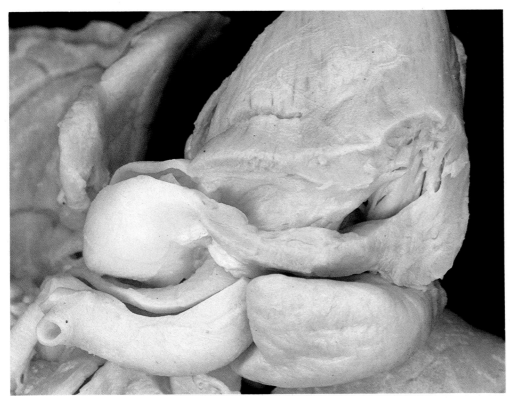

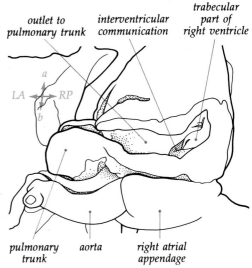

Fig. 7.2 *Rudimentary right ventricle with double inlet left ventricle and ventriculoarterial concordance ('Holmes heart'), surgically orientated. By courtesy of Dr. J.R. Zuberbuhler.*

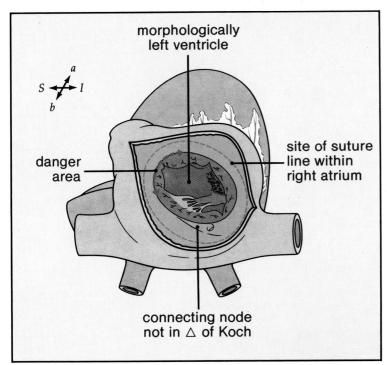

Fig. 7.3 *Position of the anomalous anterior node in double inlet left ventricle seen through the right atrium. The suggested suture line for closing the valve (if required) would avoid the node whatever its precise position.*

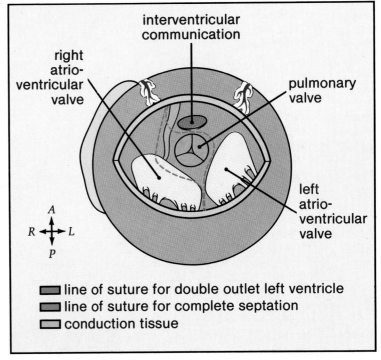

Fig. 7.4 *Option for septation in double inlet left ventricle considered relative to the conduction tissue distribution, as seen through an apical 'fishmouth' incision in the left ventricle. Compare with Fig. 7.1.*

defect (Fig. 7.1). The suture line securing this patch must cross the conduction tissue axis. The only method of septation which avoids the conduction tissues places the patch well to the right of the pulmonary outflow tract, producing double outlet from the newly created left ventricle. This necessitates closure of the pulmonary trunk and construction of an extracardiac conduit. The Mayo Clinic Group pioneered septation using this approach (*McGoon et al., 1977*) but have now abandoned it in favour of the modified Fontan procedure (*Gale et al., 1979*). Pacifico and his colleagues (1983) still favour septation and accept the likelihood of producing heart block by placing the patch as shown in Fig. 7.4. Here the anomalous node is located anterior to the right atrioventricular orifice (Fig. 7.3) and the penetrating bundle lies alongside the pulmonary annulus. The long penetrating bundle then runs superior to the pulmonary valve and crosses above the inter-ventricular communication when seen through a right-sided or 'fishmouth' ventriculotomy (Fig. 7.4). In its course above the interventricular communication the non-branching bundle is relatively narrow and it is theoretically possible to place sutures to either side of it, thus reducing the risk of heart block. However, the problem is to identify the bundle precisely. It can certainly be seen with the 'eye of faith' in the fixed heart but only experience will show if this is possible in the living. Some authorities have also suggested septation through an atriotomy.

An impression of the conduction tissues seen through this approach is illustrated in Fig. 7.5. Another prerequisite for successful septation is a heart of a reasonable size (*Stefanelli et al., 1984*). It may be necessary initially to band the pulmonary trunk if there is no naturally occurring pulmonary stenosis. This carries the recognized risk of inducing ventricular hypertrophy and severe stenosis of the interventricular communication (*Freedom et al., 1977*). If resection of a restrictive interventricular communication is necessary, it is the right-hand and inferior margin which should be removed when the approach is from the left ventricle. If approached through a left-sided rudimentary right ventricle, the resection should be towards the apical and superior parts of the interventricular communication (Fig. 7.6).

To the best of our knowledge, very few cases of double inlet right ventricle have undergone corrective surgery. They, too, should be amenable to a modified Fontan procedure, while septation is not impossible (*Girod et al., 1984*). Almost always there is a rudimentary left ventricle present, but it will rarely (if ever) be possible to incorporate this into the postseptation circulatory patterns. The trabecular septum in these cases does extend to the crux and, thus, there is a normally located conduction system, except on the rare occasion when the rudimentary left ventricle is right-sided (*Essed et al., 1980*).

Double inlet indeterminate ventricle has infrequently been septated with success (*Hamilton, Arnold & Wilkinson, 1978*). It is important to distinguish double inlet to a sole indeterminate ventricle from a huge ventricular septal defect. Septation of the latter anomaly will be a formidable surgical undertaking, but the remnant of the ventricular septum does provide a landmark for placement of the patch, remembering that the conduction axis will be posteriorly placed as in an atrioventricular septal defect (see Chapter 6, iii). In double inlet to a sole indeterminate ventricle there is no such guide for septation. Indeed, the common apical trabecular portion is usually criss-crossed by large trabeculae and it is rare to find a discrete plane of cleavage between the atrioventricular valves (Fig. 7.7). Septation is a considerable procedure with the added problem of the bizarre disposition of the conduction tissue (*Wilkinson et al., 1976*). If the haemodynamic criteria are fulfilled, a modified Fontan procedure may be another option, in which case, when closing the right atrioventricular valve, the likeliest landmarks to the connecting atrioventricular node are as described for double inlet left ventricle.

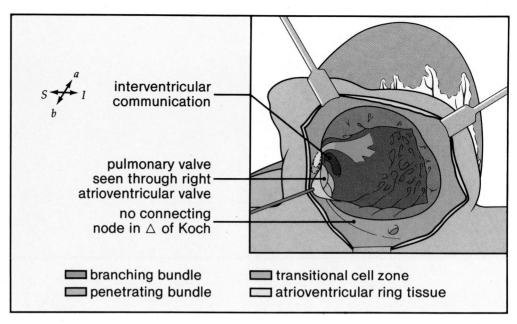

Fig. 7.5 *Conduction tissue distribution in double inlet left ventricle with left-sided rudimentary right ventricle and ventriculoarterial discordance as seen through the right atrioventricular valve.*

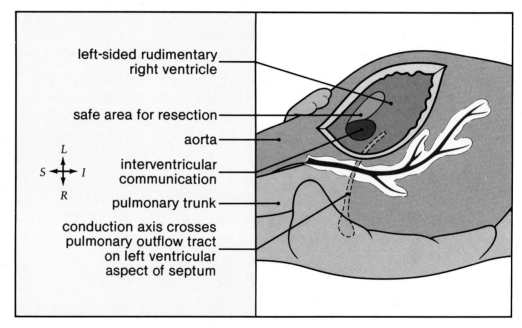

Fig. 7.6 *Relationship of the conduction axis to the interventricular communication seen from the rudimentary right ventricle with univentricular atrioventricular connexion to a left ventricle.*

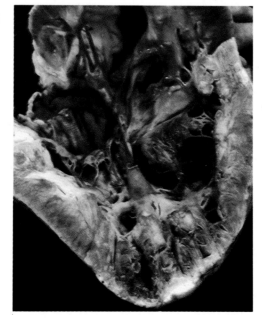

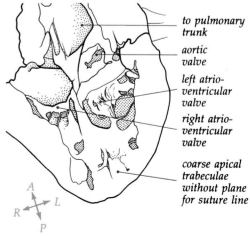

Fig. 7.7 *Double inlet and double outlet from a solitary indeterminate ventricle in anatomical orientation.*

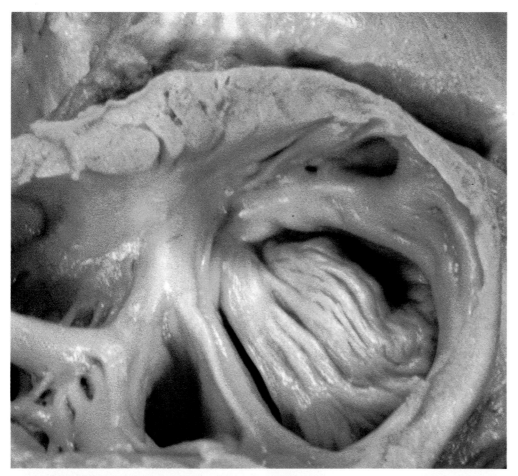

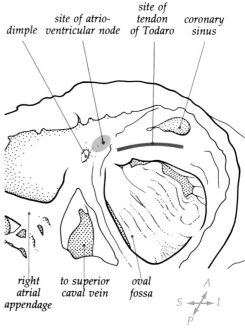

site of atrio-
dimple ventricular node

site of
tendon
of Todaro coronary
sinus

right
atrial
appendage

to superior
caval vein

oval
fossa

A
S ← → I
P

Fig. 7.8 *Right atrial morphology with 'classical' tricuspid atresia seen in surgical orientation. Note the absence of any tricuspid valve annulus. The site of the atrioventricular node has been superimposed.*

delimiting
left
coronary
artery

rudimentary
ventricle

right
atrial
appendage

right
bundle
branch

L
S ← → I
R

right
coronary
artery

delimiting
right marginal
coronary
artery

aorta

inter-
ventricular
communication

Fig. 7.9 *Operative view of rudimentary right ventricle with classical tricuspid atresia: (left) external appearances; the right delimiting artery descends at the acute margin of the atrioventricular junction; (right) internal morphology.*

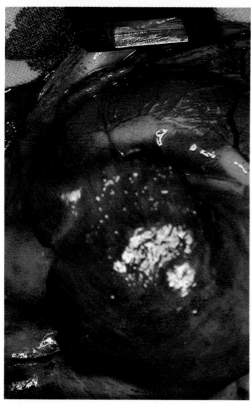

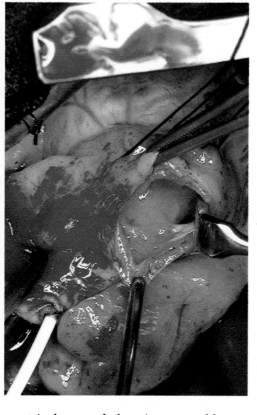

ii. Absent atrioventricular connexion

Although frequently the anatomy is not fully appreciated, most examples of classical tricuspid atresia have complete absence of their right atrioventricular connexion (see Chapter 5, Fig. 5.5) while a good proportion of cases of mitral atresia have absence of the left atrioventricular connexion (see Fig. 5.6). Therefore, their

ventricular morphology is comparable to hearts with double inlet since the atria connect to only one ventricle. It is also true that the variations of segmental combinations are just as great for absent connexion as for double inlet ventricle. However, by far the greatest number of cases encountered have the classical types of valve atresia and we will concentrate attention on these.

Usually in tricuspid atresia the morphologically right atrium is blind-ending and has no vestige of tricuspid valve tissue in its floor (Fig. 7.8). Because of the absent right atrioventricular connexion the right ventricle is rudimentary (Fig. 7.9), lacking an inlet portion. The trabecular part of the right ventricle is separated from the left ventricle by the apical trabecular septum

7.5

which, as in double inlet left ventricle, does not extend to the crux (Fig. 7.10). The determinant of surgical options is the ventriculoarterial connexion. Usually this is concordant and the rudimentary right ventricle can then be incorporated into the pulmonary circulation using the modified Fontan procedure (*Henry et al., 1974*). From the standpoint of atrial surgery, the muscle bundles should be disturbed as little as possible since the right atrium is to become the major pumping chamber for the pulmonary circulation. The sinus node and its blood supply should be avoided as atrial arrhythmia is a recognized life-threatening postoperative complication. The need for caval valves is still not resolved, but some patients can do without them. However, whenever a well formed Eustachian valve is encountered (a frequent occurrence), it should be preserved. After the rudimentary right ventricle has been incorporated into the circulation, it is necessary to close the interventricular communication. This can usually be done safely since the conduction tissue is carried on the left ventricular aspect of the septum well away from the crest (Fig. 7.11).

When there is ventriculoarterial discordance (transposition) with tricuspid atresia, it is not possible to incorporate the rudimentary right ventricle into the pulmonary circuit. If a Fontan procedure is to be performed, a direct right atrial to pulmonary trunk anastomosis is required. This can also be done with a conduit (*Doty et al., 1981*). Should resection of the margins of the interventricular communication be necessary in cases with aortic obstruction, it must be remembered that the conduction tissue runs on the left ventricular aspect of the septum, postero-inferior to the interventricular communication except in those rare cases where the communication is atretic and an apical trabecular defect is present (Fig. 7.11).

In rare cases, tricuspid atresia may be due to an imperforate valve membrane interposed between the right atrium and ventricle, but only very rarely will the membrane be of a size sufficient to permit resection and insertion of a prosthesis. In these cases it is important to distinguish them from classical tricuspid atresia (*Scalia et al., 1984*).

In a great majority of cases, mitral atresia is not amenable to surgical treatment because of its association with aortic atresia. Early palliative procedures for this lesion are very much at an experimental stage (*Doty & Knott, 1977; Norwood, Kirklin & Sanders, 1980*). Nonetheless, it is worth noting that some success has been achieved in providing 'correction' using a modified Fontan procedure (*Norwood, Lang & Hansen, 1983*). In some cases of 'mitral' atresia, however, the aortic outflow tract is patent.

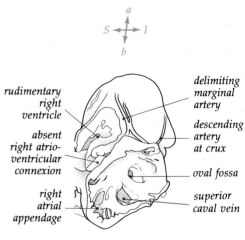

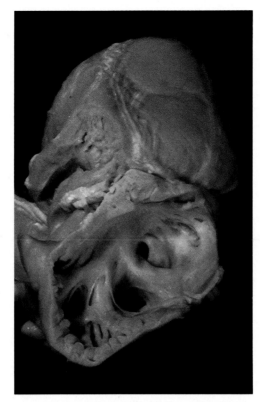

Fig. 7.10 *Surgically orientated view from the right and behind showing how the septum in classical tricuspid atresia does not extend to the crux. The delimiting artery descends at the acute margin.*

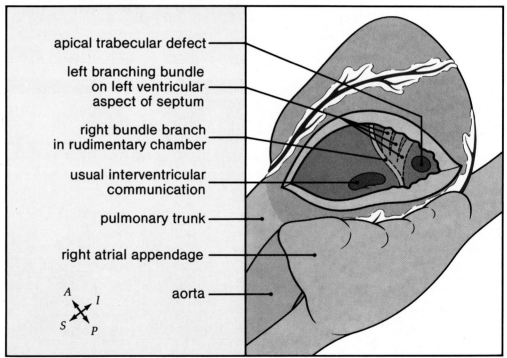

apical trabecular defect

left branching bundle on left ventricular aspect of septum

right bundle branch in rudimentary chamber

usual interventricular communication

pulmonary trunk

right atrial appendage

aorta

Fig. 7.11 *Relationship of the conduction axis to the usual interventricular communication and to an apical trabecular defect in classical tricuspid atresia.*

It is questionable whether all of these should be termed 'mitral atresia' since in many the embryological considerations suggest that the left connexion, had it formed, would have been guarded by a tricuspid valve. Irrespective of such speculation, all cases have an absent left-sided atrioventricular connexion so that pulmonary venous return has no route to the ventricles other than by way of an atrial septal defect and the right atrioventricular valve. Initial survival in these cases therefore depends on the state of the atrial septum, and the operation of choice is likely to be a Blalock-Hanlon

septostomy (*Mickell et al., 1980*), after which some sort of modified Fontan procedure may be possible. In a heart where the right atrium connected to the left ventricle and there was an anterior rudimentary right ventricle and ventriculoarterial concordance, it proved possible to channel the left atrium to the left ventricle and aorta and to place a conduit from the isolated right atrium to the rudimentary right ventricle and pulmonary trunk (*Shore et al., 1982*). Such cases are exceedingly rare and, overall, the prospects of corrective surgery are not good.

iii. Complete transposition

This malformation is characterized by the atria being connected to their appropriate ventricles but with inappropriate ventriculoarterial connexions. The result is atrioventricular concordance and ventriculoarterial discordance. Some refer to this combination simply as 'transposition' or 'TGA', but there is controversy surrounding the use of this term (*Tynan & Anderson, 1979*). This is in part because many use 'transposition' only to describe a discordant ventriculo-arterial connexion (*Van Praagh et al., 1971*) while others use the term to describe any heart with an anterior aorta (*Van Mierop, 1971*). Those who use the term 'TGA' to describe a discordant ventriculoarterial connexion do not restrict it to the setting of atrioventricular concordance. 'Transposition', when defined simply as a discordant ventriculoarterial connexion, can clearly coexist with double inlet ventricle or absent connexion, and it is these latter anomalies which then become the dominant features. There is, therefore, a need for a term which describes only the chamber combinations of atrioventricular concordance and ventriculoarterial discordance (Fig. 7.12). Our preference is to use the term 'complete transposition'. There has been a vogue for using 'd-transposition' to the same end, but this does not accurately describe those cases with the usual atrial arrangement, atrioventricular concordance, ventriculoarterial discordance and left-sided aorta. Neither does 'd-transposition' describe that majority of patients with these chamber combinations and mirror-image atrial arrangement. It should also be noted that complete transposition as defined here refers only to patients with lateralized atria (usual and mirror-image arrangements). When ventriculoarterial discordance occurs in the setting of atrial isomerism, it is the venous and atrioventricular junctional anomalies which usually dominate the anatomical and clinical considerations, so these cases are also excluded from our category of complete transposition.

From the surgical standpoint, the two major subgroups of complete transposition are those without any major additional complicating lesions (simple complete transposition) and those with additional malformations (complex complete transposition). We will deal with the morphological aspects of the complicating anomalies in turn, but the atrial anatomy is comparable within the whole group.

Though an arterial switch procedure is clearly feasible in selected cases, operations designed to redirect venous blood at the atrial level predominate in world-wide experience. When planning these operations, the disposition of the cardiac nodes and their blood supply is an important factor. The presence of

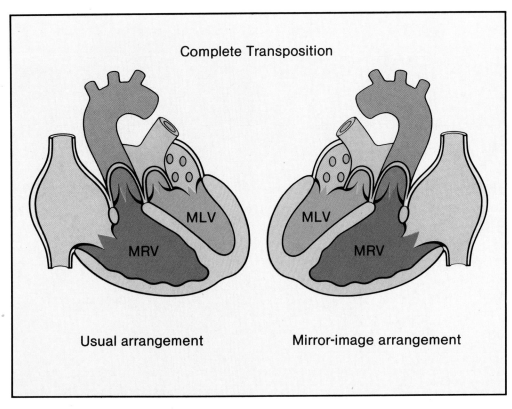

Fig. 7.12 *The segmental combinations which produce complete transposition.*

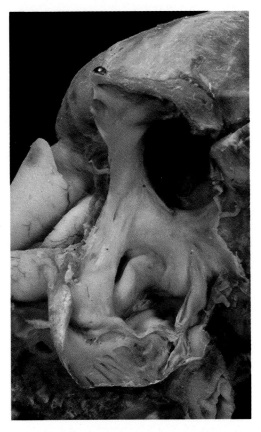

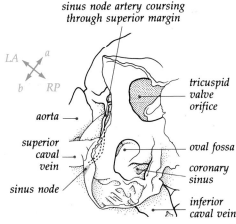

Fig. 7.13 *Relation of the sinus node artery to the atrial septum in complete transposition in surgical orientation.*

ventriculoarterial discordance does not in any way affect the position of the sinus node so the rules enunciated for nodal avoidance in Chapter 2 are equally applicable in complete transposition. The entire terminal sulcus should be avoided as the sinus node may occupy a 'horseshoe' position over the crest of the superior caval-right atrial junction, although it is usually in a lateral position (see Fig. 2.7). Furthermore, the nodal artery may enter the sulcus across the

crest of the appendage or after running a retrocaval course (see Fig. 2.8, left). Of more importance is the course taken by the nodal artery as it ascends the interatrial groove. The artery frequently burrows into the atrial musculature, running within the superior border of the oval fossa (Fig. 7.13) where it is at risk when incising the septum for a Senning or Mustard procedure, or during a Blalock-Hanlon septostomy.

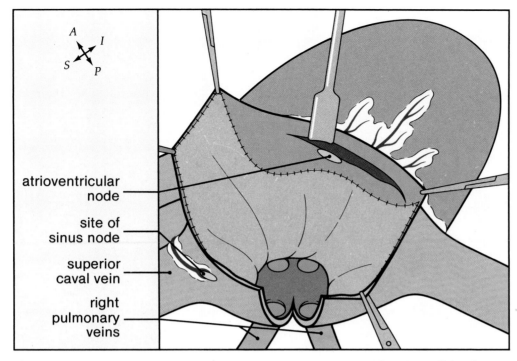

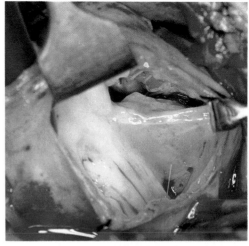

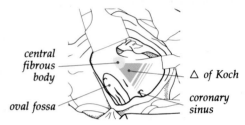

atrioventricular
node

site of
sinus node

superior
caval vein

right
pulmonary
veins

Fig. 7.14 *Incision which widens the new pulmonary venous atrium without jeopardizing the sinus node in Mustard's operation.*

central
fibrous
body

oval fossa

△ of Koch

coronary
sinus

Fig. 7.15 *Operative view of the landmarks to the triangle of Koch.*

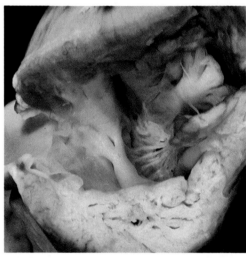

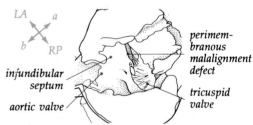

LA   a

b   RP

infundibular
septum

aortic valve

perimem-
branous
malalignment
defect

tricuspid
valve

Fig. 7.16 *Outlet malalignment defect in complete transposition which extends to become perimembranous, seen in surgical orientation.*

It is well to keep in mind certain key considerations when carrying out a venous switch procedure. They include cannulation of the superior caval vein a good distance from the cavoatrial junction, incising the right atrium well clear of the terminal sulcus and avoiding traction, suction or suturing in the area of the superior border of the sulcus. If an incision is required across the sulcus to widen the newly constructed pulmonary venous atrium in Mustard's operation, it can be made between the right pulmonary veins without fear of damaging the sinus node or artery (Fig. 7.14).

This entire discussion is highly pertinent to various considerations regarding the genesis of arrhythmias after Mustard's operation. It has been suggested that the arrhythmias are due to damage to the so-called 'specialized internodal pathways' (*Isaacson et al., 1972*). Although, as we explained in Chapter 2, there are no such pathways composed of histologically specialized tissue, the atrioventricular impulse is preferentially conducted from the sinus node through the thicker muscles of the right atrial wall and septum. It is advantageous, therefore, to preserve at least one of these routes. If the terminal crest is to be divided to enlarge the new pulmonary venous atrium, this is a further reason to preserve the superior border of the oval fossa. These procedures, together with scrupulous avoidance of the sinus node and its blood supply, mean that arrhythmias can be virtually abolished after Mustard's operation (*Ullal, Anderson & Lincoln, 1979*), taking into account arrhythmias which were present prior to operation (*Southall et al., 1980*). Considerations of sinus node disposition

and arterial supply are equally important in Senning's operation, when these areas are just as much at risk as during Mustard's procedure.

It is always important to avoid the atrioventricular node. The landmarks to this vital structure are the same as in the normal heart (Fig. 7.15); so, providing all surgery is performed outside the triangle of Koch, injury to the node will be avoided. The technique of cutting back the coronary sinus should be carefully considered. It is possible to perform this procedure without damaging the node and its transitional cell zones, but the incision will undoubtedly cross one of the preferential routes of conduction. For this reason it is safer to place the inferior suture line so as to avoid completely the triangle of Koch.

The major complicating lesion in complete transposition is the presence of a ventricular septal defect with or without left ventricular outflow tract obstruction. Any other lesion can coexist if anatomically possible and the anatomy will then be as described for the lesion in isolation.

A ventricular septal defect in complete transposition can be as variable in morphology as those found in isolation (see Chapter 6, ii). The majority of defects are in the outlet portions of the ventricular mass and have their own peculiar characteristics. They can either be perimembranous (Fig. 7.16) or have a muscular posteroinferior rim (Fig. 7.17). The distinguishing feature between the two is whether or not the posterior limb of the septomarginal trabecula fuses with the ventriculoinfundibular fold. If there is fusion (Fig. 7.17), the conduction tissues will be buttressed and there will be

pulmonary-tricuspid valve discontinuity. If there is no fusion, the defect will be perimembranous and there will be fibrous continuity between the pulmonary and tricuspid valves. The penetrating bundle will be at risk in this area of fibrous continuity (Fig. 7.16).

These defects have other features of surgical significance. The tension apparatus of the tricuspid valve tends to

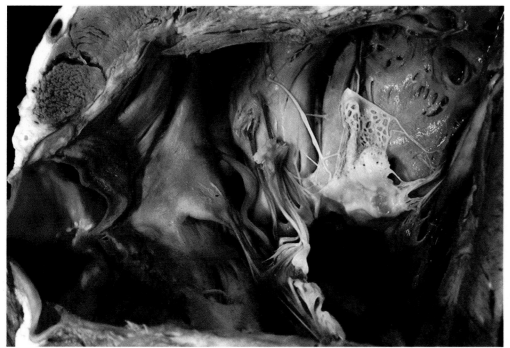

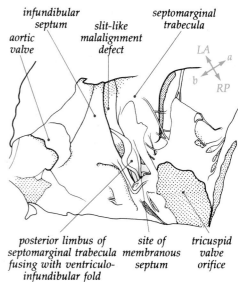

infundibular
septum
aortic
valve
slit-like
malalignment
defect
septomarginal
trabecula

LA
a
b
RP

posterior limbus of
septomarginal trabecula
fusing with ventriculo-
infundibular fold
site of
membranous
septum
tricuspid
valve
orifice

Fig. 7.17 *Muscular outlet malalignment defect in complete transposition seen in surgical orientation from the right ventricle.*

course over the defect and attach to the outlet septum or to the ventriculo-infundibular fold (Fig. 7.17). This makes closure of the defect difficult without damage to the tricuspid valve. This is of particular significance as the valve will be subjected to systemic pressures after a venous redirection procedure. Also, the borders of the defect diverge towards the parietal and anterior heart walls. In hearts with ventriculoarterial concordance, the anterior margin of a ventricular septal defect is usually well circumscribed. In these cases with complete transposition, the outlet septum becomes malaligned in relation to the trabecular septum as it inserts into the anterior wall of the right ventricular outflow tract. The defect is therefore more difficult to close at this anterior margin.

Inlet defects, either perimembranous or muscular, also have surgical significance. Should a Rastelli procedure be considered for a patient with this type of defect and coexisting pulmonary stenosis, there will be difficulty in connecting the defect to the aorta. Apical or multiple muscular defects also present this disadvantage for intraventricular rerouting to the aorta. Perimembranous inlet defects, sometimes incorrectly termed 'atrioventricular canal defects', are the harbingers of a straddling tricuspid valve, which should always be suspected when the right ventricle is hypoplastic. A straddling valve increases markedly the risks of surgery, not least because of the abnormal disposition of the conduction tissues (see Chapter 6, iv).

Subpulmonary obstruction in complete transposition can be produced by any lesion which would produce subaortic obstruction in the normal heart. Rarer lesions, such as anomalous insertion of the tension apparatus of the atrio-ventricular valve, are probably beyond

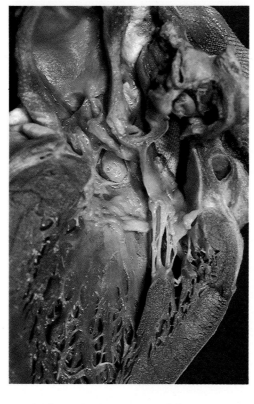

surgical repair. Aneurysm of the membranous septum or similar fibrous tissue 'tags' should be readily amenable to removal, although a subpulmonary fibrous diaphragm poses more problems as it directly overlies the left bundle branch (Fig. 7.18). The difficulties are compounded when the fibrous obstruction is more extensive, because then it can form a subvalvar tunnel. The other quadrants of the outflow tract are also vulnerable because of their proximity to the left coronary artery or because they are formed by leaflets of the mitral valve. The safest area for resection, then, is beneath the remnant of the left margin of the ventriculoinfundibular fold (*Wilcox, Henry & Anderson, 1983*). When subpulmonary obstruction coexists with a

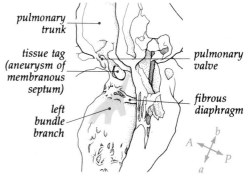

pulmonary
trunk
tissue tag
(aneurysm of
membranous
septum)
left
bundle
branch
pulmonary
valve
fibrous
diaphragm

A
b
P
a

Fig. 7.18 *Anatomically orientated left ventricular outflow tract in complete transposition with discrete diaphragmatic obstruction together with a fibrous tag. The site of the vulnerable left bundle branch has been superimposed. The safe area is the part of the outflow tract immediately beneath the ventriculoinfundibular fold.*

ventricular septal defect, there is almost always posterior deviation and insertion of the outlet septum into the left ventricle. This usually means that the aortic valve overrides the septum with a good-sized defect, which is favourable for a Rastelli procedure. Should the defect be restrictive and a Rastelli operation is still desirable, it is possible to resect safely the outlet septum, which never harbours conduction tissue. Should the defect be situated other than in the ventricular outlets, the chances of successfully accomplishing a Rastelli procedure are considerably reduced. It should also be remembered that valvar pulmonary stenosis frequently accompanies subvalvar stenosis.

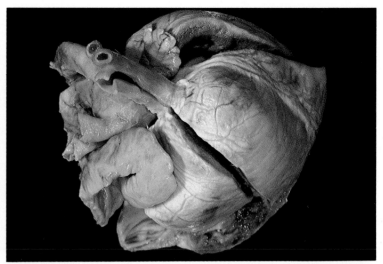

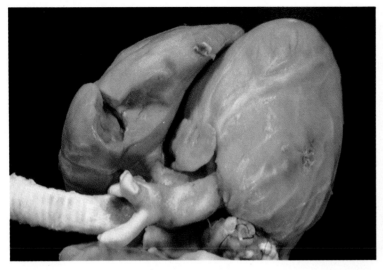

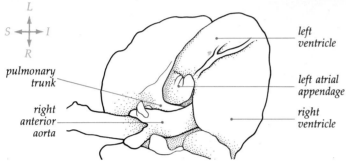

Fig. 7.19 *Usual anterior and right-sided aortic position found in complete transposition, seen in surgical orientation.*

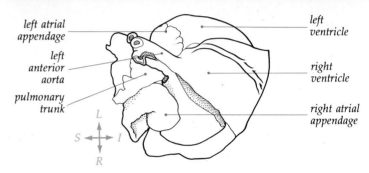

Fig. 7.20 *Less common arrangement in complete transposition with aorta in left anterior position together with the usual arrangement of atrial chambers, seen in surgical orientation.*

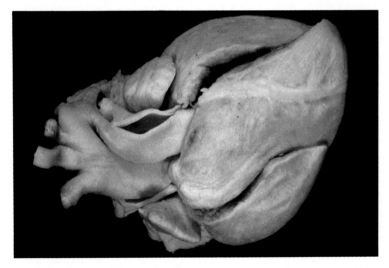

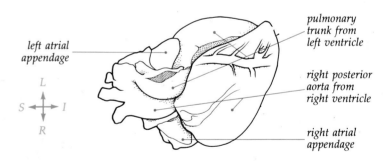

Fig. 7.21 *Rare arrangement in complete transposition where the aorta is found in right-sided and posterior position ('normal relations'), seen in surgical orientation.*

Thus far we have devoted attention exclusively to the segmental anatomy of complete transposition. There is, of course, further variation in terms of both arterial relationships and infundibular anatomy. These variations do not alter the intracardiac anatomy and are therefore of relatively minor surgical significance. For example, the aorta is usually anterior and to the right in complete transposition (Fig. 7.19) but, in some cases, the aorta may be anterior and to the left (Fig. 7.20) and, in rare cases, may be posterior and to the right of the pulmonary trunk (Fig. 7.21). As suggested, these different relationships do not alter the basic anatomy; but they do show why it is inadvisable

to use the term 'd-transposition' for the group as a whole when a patient with a left-sided aorta must have 'l-transposition'.

There are some clues to associated lesions to be drawn from these unexpected arterial relationships. With a left-sided aorta, there is a high incidence of doubly-committed subarterial ventricular septal defects (*Lincoln et al., 1976*), an arrangement convenient for connexion of the aorta to the left ventricle and Rastelli's procedure. When the aorta is posterior, there is usually a subpulmonary infundibulum with the aortic valve in fibrous continuity with the mitral valve through the roof of a perimembranous

septal defect (*Van Praagh et al., 1971; Wilkinson et al., 1975; Arteaga et al., 1981*). This unusual anatomy can create difficulty both at initial diagnosis and at subsequent surgery. More recently, cases with a posterior aorta have been observed with an intact ventricular septum (*Buchler, Bembom & Buchler, 1984*). Variations in infundibular morphology in themselves are unlikely to give problems. The expected subaortic muscular infundibulum in the right ventricle is most frequently encountered with pulmonary-mitral fibrous continuity in the left ventricle. Rarely, there may be a complete muscular infundibulum in both ventricles while even more rarely, as

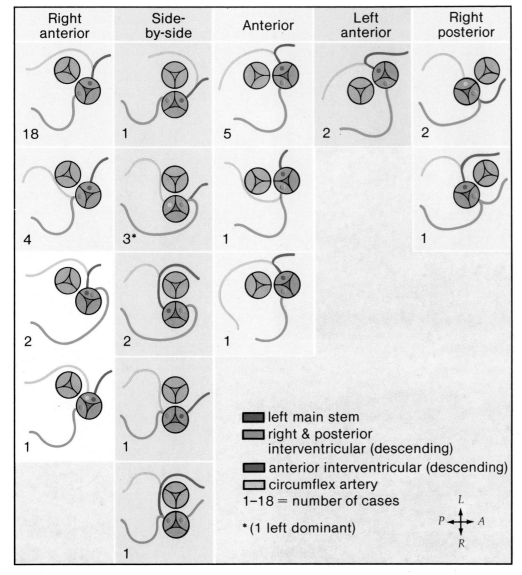

Right anterior	Side-by-side	Anterior	Left anterior	Right posterior
18	1	5	2	2
4	3*	1		1
2	2	1		
1	1			
	1			

■ left main stem
□ right & posterior interventricular (descending)
■ anterior interventricular (descending)
□ circumflex artery
1–18 = number of cases
*(1 left dominant)

L
P ←→ A
R

Fig. 7.22 *Arrangements of the origins of the coronary arteries in complete transposition. The patterns in the yellow boxes are those most likely to give problems to the surgeon during 'arterial switch' procedure. Based on the original concept of Mrs. A. Smith.*

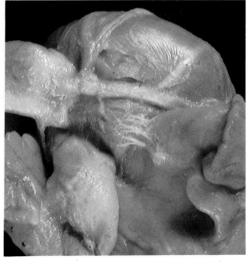

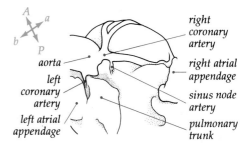

A
a
b
P

aorta — right coronary artery
left coronary artery — right atrial appendage
left atrial appendage — sinus node artery
pulmonary trunk

Fig. 7.23 *Origins of the coronary arteries in typical complete transposition are adjacent to the pulmonary trunk and are close to the origin of the sinus node artery.*

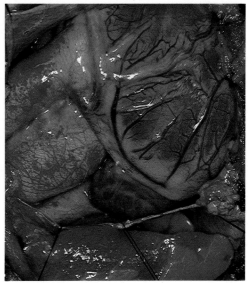

L
S ←→ I
R

aorta — anomalous origin of anterior interventricular coronary artery
pulmonary artery — right coronary artery
superior caval vein

Fig. 7.24 *Operative view of complete transposition with left-sided aorta and anomalous origin of the anterior interventricular from the right coronary artery. If necessary, the arterial origin could be easily 'switched' to the pulmonary root.*

described above, there may be a subpulmonary infundibulum with aortic-mitral continuity when the transposed aorta is in posterior position.

The final feature of surgical importance in complete transposition is the coronary arterial morphology, particularly in view of the feasibility of the arterial switch procedure for operative correction. This operation involves transecting the ascending aorta and pulmonary trunk and reconnecting them to the appropriate ventricles. There have been procedures advocated which permit reconnexion without coronary artery translocation using ingenious window techniques (*Aubert et al., 1978*) or more complicated conduit procedures (*Damus, Thomson & McLoughlin, 1982; Stansel, 1975; Kaye, 1975*). The more popular option is to transpose the arterial trunks and the coronary arteries (*Jatene et al., 1976; Yacoub & Radley-Smith, 1978*), which is favoured by the coronary arterial anatomy (Fig. 7.22). Almost invariably

the coronary arteries arise from the aortic sinuses facing the pulmonary trunk (*Gittenberger-de Groot et al., 1983*), so that the coronary arterial origins are transferred across a relatively short distance (Fig. 7.23). This rule stands whatever the relationship of the aorta to the pulmonary trunk (Fig. 7.22). Unusual features which may compromise this transfer are largely related to an anomalous course of the coronary arteries themselves in relation to the vascular pedicle (Fig. 7.24) (*Rowlatt, 1962; Shaher & Puddu, 1966*). However, in the opinion of Yacoub and Radley-Smith (1978), these variations are unlikely to give problems. What may be more significant is that sometimes the origin of the sinus node artery is very close to the origin of the coronary artery from the aorta. In these circumstances, transfer of the coronary artery may traumatize or destroy the sinus node artery. Otherwise, thus far, there is no evidence of postoperative rhythm problems with the switch procedure.

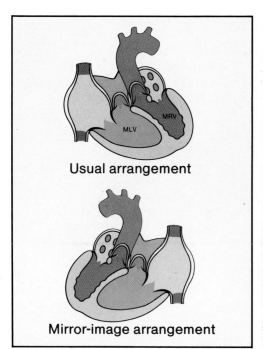

Usual arrangement

Mirror-image arrangement

Fig. 7.25 *The segmental combinations which produce congenitally corrected transposition.*

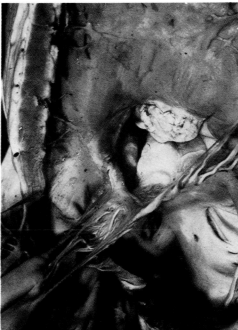

Fig. 7.26 *Apical view of the right-sided morphologically left ventricle, surgically orientated to show the anomalous conduction tissue axis. By courtesy of Prof. A.E. Becker.*

aneurysmal interventricular
membranous septum

anterior
conduction
tissue
axis

pulmonary
valve

mitral
valve
septal
leaflet

anterior
papillary
muscle

anterior recess of
morphologically left ventricle

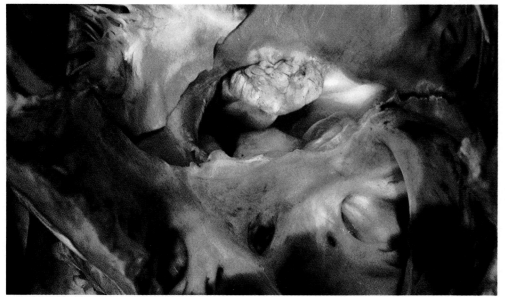

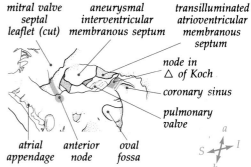

mitral valve
septal
leaflet (cut)

aneurysmal
interventricular
membranous septum

transilluminated
atrioventricular
membranous
septum

node in
△ of Koch

coronary sinus

pulmonary
valve

atrial
appendage

anterior
node

oval
fossa

Fig. 7.27 *Right atrioventricular junction in congenitally corrected transposition, same heart as in Fig. 7.26, in surgical orientation. The septal attachment of the mitral valve has been removed to show the malalignment gap and the anomalous distribution of the conduction tissues. By courtesy of Prof. A.E. Becker.*

iv. Congenitally corrected transposition

We use the term 'congenitally corrected transposition' to describe the combination of atrioventricular discordance and ventriculoarterial discordance. This term has a long pedigree, but of late there has been a vogue for replacing it with 'l-transposition', which suffers from the same problem as 'd-transposition'. Not all cases of corrected transposition have a left-sided aorta while not all cases of 'l-transposition' have the combination of atrioventricular discordance and ventriculoarterial discordance. Hence, our preference is to use 'congenitally corrected transposition' to describe this specific segmental combination. It can exist with atria in the usual arrangement or mirror-image atria (Fig. 7.25), but not with atrial isomerism.

To comprehend fully the complexities of corrected transposition one must be aware that the essential feature of this lesion is malalignment between the inlet part of the ventricular septum and the atrial septum (*Losekoot et al., 1983*). At the crux the two septa are in line, but when traced forwards they diverge markedly. This produces a malalignment gap. Into this gap the subpulmonary outflow tract from the morphologically left ventricle is wedged (Fig. 7.26). This abnormal anatomy accounts for the single most important surgical feature of corrected transposition, namely the unusual disposition of the atrioventricular conduction tissues. Because of the malalignment gap it is not possible for the normal atrioventricular node at the apex of the triangle of Koch to penetrate the fibrous annulus and make contact with the ventricular conduction tissues. Instead, an anomalous atrioventricular node, found in an anterolateral position as in double inlet left ventricle (see Fig. 7.3),

gives rise to a penetrating atrioventricular bundle. This bundle penetrates the atrioventricular tissue plane lateral to the area of pulmonary-mitral fibrous continuity (Fig. 7.27). A long non-branching bundle then runs round the anterior quadrants of the pulmonary valve annulus, crossing the characteristic anterior recess of the morphologically left ventricle before descending onto the trabecular septum and branching in mirror-image fashion. The fan-like left bundle branch is distributed in the right-sided morphologically left ventricle while the cord-like right bundle branch penetrates the septum to reach the left-sided morphologically right ventricle (*Anderson et al., 1974*). The transposed aorta typically arises from this morphologically right ventricle above a complete muscular infundibulum and usually in a left-sided position (Fig. 7.28).

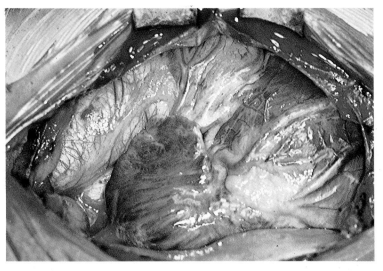

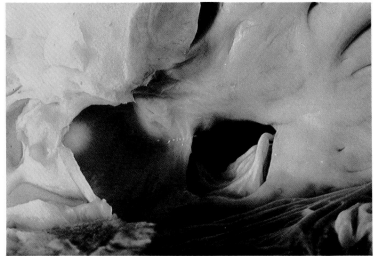

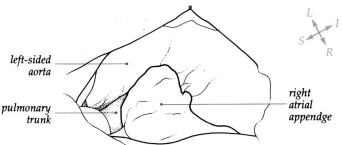

left-sided
aorta

pulmonary
trunk

right
atrial
appendge

L
I
S
R

Fig. 7.28 *Operative view showing the typical left-sided position of the aorta in congenitally corrected transposition. By courtesy of Dr. J Quaegebeur, University of Leiden, The Netherlands.*

A
b ← → *a*
P

dome-shaped
pulmonary
valve stenosis

perimem-
branous inlet
ventricular
septal defect

anterior recess

anterior
conduction
tissue axis

morpho-
logically
tricuspid
valve seen
through defect

mitral valve

Fig. 7.29 *Morphologically left ventricular aspect of a perimembranous defect in congenitally corrected transposition seen in surgical orientation. By courtesy of Prof. A.E. Becker.*

When corrected transposition exists without any other anomaly, the circulation of the blood is normal. Unfortunately this situation is very much the exception (*Losekoot et al., 1983*). Usually one or more of three associated lesions are found, namely ventricular septal defect, pulmonary stenosis and left-sided atrioventricular valve anomalies. Not surprisingly these lesions often require surgical treatment.

A ventricular septal defect is present in about seventy percent of cases. It may be perimembranous, muscular or subarterial, as in the heart with normal connexions, but is usually of the perimembranous inlet type. Then, because of the wedge position of the pulmonary valve, the pulmonary trunk tends to override the defect (Fig. 7.29). When seen from the right atrium, it is shielded by the anterior commissure of the right-sided mitral valve (Fig. 7.30). While closing the defect it is vital to bear in mind the abnormal position of the atrioventricular node in the region of the anterior commissure with the non-branching atrioventricular bundle. The regular node at the apex of the triangle of Koch is also present but hardly ever gives rise to a penetrating bundle (Fig. 7.30). Instead, the bundle arises from the anomalous anterolateral node, penetrates the area of pulmonary-mitral valvar continuity and then runs round the subpulmonary outflow tract to descend on the anterosuperior margin of the defect (Fig. 7.31).

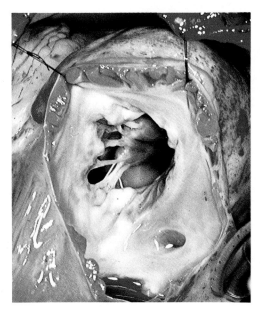

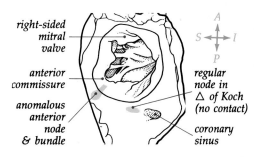

right-sided
mitral
valve

anterior
commissure

anomalous
anterior
node
& bundle

regular
node in
△ of Koch
(no contact)

coronary
sinus

A
S ← → *I*
P

Fig. 7.30 *Operative view of the opened right atrium in congenitally corrected transposition with perimembranous inlet defect to show the position of the anomalous anterior node. By courtesy of Dr. J. Quaegebeur.*

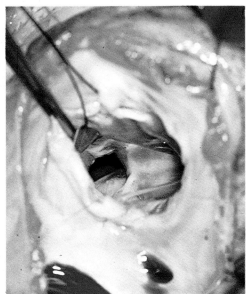

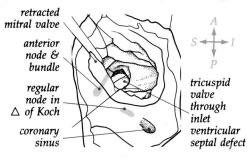

retracted
mitral valve

anterior
node &
bundle

regular
node in
△ of Koch

coronary
sinus

tricuspid
valve
through
inlet
ventricular
septal defect

A
S ← → *I*
P

Fig. 7.31 *Retracted mitral valve of the heart shown in Fig. 7.30 to show the perimembranous defect. By courtesy of Dr. J. Quaegebeur.*

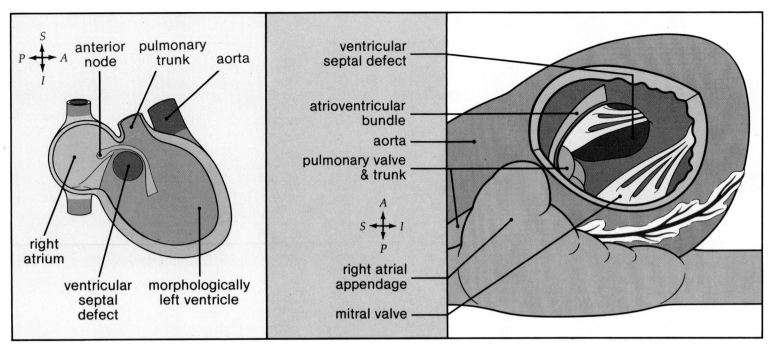

Fig. 7.32 *Illustration of the difficulty in showing simply the relationship of the conduction axis to the pulmonary valve in congenitally corrected transposition (left). The correct course can only be seen in a drawing which provides perspective (right).*

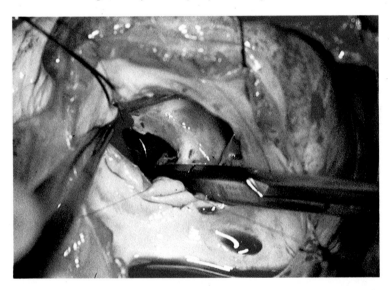

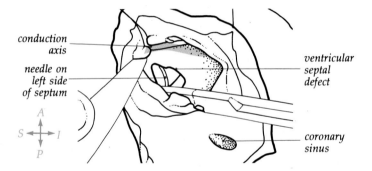

Fig. 7.33 *When closing the defect shown in Fig. 7.31, the stitches are placed on the morphologically right ventricular aspect of the septum, that is on the left side. By courtesy of Dr. J. Quaegebeur.*

Several observers have suggested that the bundle runs between the pulmonary valve and the defect within the outlet septum (*Stewart, Manning & Siegel, 1977; Kupersmith et al., 1974*). We have never seen a bundle in this position, nor has one been mapped in this site during the extensive experience with this condition at the Mayo Clinic (*Anderson et al., 1978; Danielson et al., 1978*). We believe that the reason the bundle is shown in this site is one of perspective. When the surgeon tries to put his observations into one dimension on paper, it is difficult not to give the impression that the bundle passes between the valve and defect (Fig. 7.32, left). It is vital to appreciate the precise anterior position of the bundle (Fig. 7.32, right).

De Leval and his colleagues (1979) suggest that the safest way to close the defect, considering its anatomy, is to place sutures on the morphologically right ventricular (left-sided) aspect (Fig. 7.33).

Although the defect invades mostly the inlet septum, it can extend to become doubly-committed and subarterial. Then, it is roofed by the conjoined aortic and pulmonary valve rings (Figs. 7.34 & 7.35). When it is perimembranous and subarterial, the conduction tissue remains in anterior position. Cases have been described, particularly in the Far East (*Okamura & Konno, 1973*), with so-called 'supracristal' defects. If such cases have a muscular inferior rim between the pulmonary and mitral valve, it is possible that the conduction axis will be posterior to the defect. We have seen a comparable case with both a perimembranous and a muscular outlet defect; the conduction axis descended the muscle bar between them. If there is doubt, it is probably wise to map the conduction tissue disposition during surgery.

As with complete transposition, any of the lesions which produce left ventricular outflow tract obstruction will produce pulmonary stenosis in congenitally corrected transposition. Valvar stenosis in isolation is rare, but it frequently coexists with subvalvar obstructive lesions. Particularly significant in this respect are fibrous tissue tags (Fig. 7.36). Fibrous diaphragmatic lesions (Fig. 7.37) or muscular obstruction are also encountered (*Anderson, Becker & Gerlis, 1975*). The overwhelming consideration in all of these types of stenosis is the presence of the non-branching bundle running round the anterior quadrants of the outflow tract (see Fig. 7.25). This makes it very difficult to resect these various lesions (apart from tags). Placement of a conduit is the safest means of avoiding postoperative heart block, although an ingenious method of avoiding the conduction tissues has been devised by Doty, Truesdell and Marvin (1983).

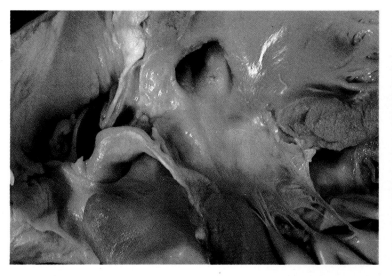

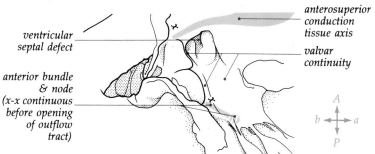

Fig. 7.34 *Morphologically left ventricular aspect of a perimembranous defect in corrected transposition which extends to become doubly-committed and subarterial, seen in surgical orientation. There is fibrous continuity of all four valves.*

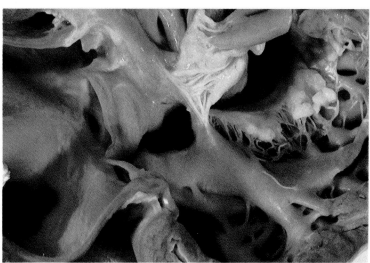

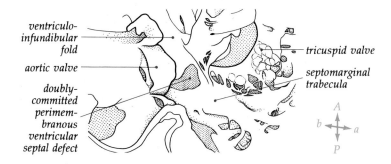

Fig. 7.35 *Left-sided morphologically right ventricular aspect of the doubly-committed defect shown in Fig. 7.34.*

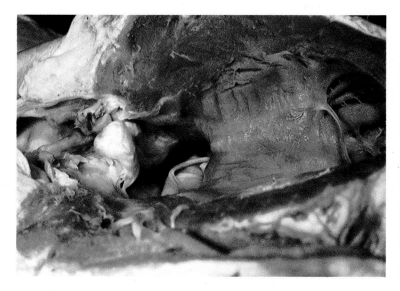

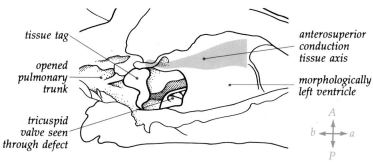

Fig. 7.36 *Subpulmonary obstruction in congenitally corrected transposition produced by a tissue tag herniated from a partially-formed membranous septum, seen in surgical orientation. By courtesy of Prof. A.E. Becker.*

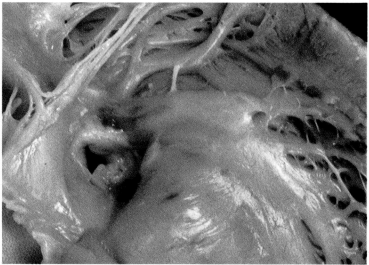

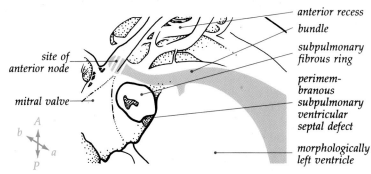

Fig. 7.37 *Subpulmonary obstruction produced by a fibrous diaphragm in corrected transposition, seen in anatomical orientation. Note the position of the conduction axis. By courtesy of Mr. Marc de Leval, Hospital for Sick Children, London.*

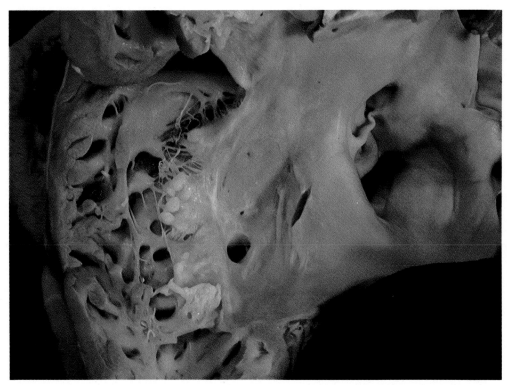

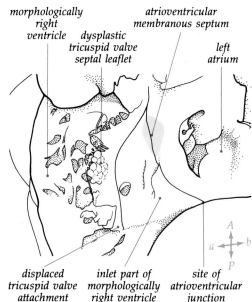

morphologically right ventricle
dysplastic tricuspid valve septal leaflet
atrioventricular membranous septum
left atrium

displaced tricuspid valve attachment
inlet part of morphologically right ventricle
site of atrioventricular junction

Fig. 7.38 *Usual form of Ebstein's malformation of the left-sided morphologically tricuspid valve found in corrected transposition.*

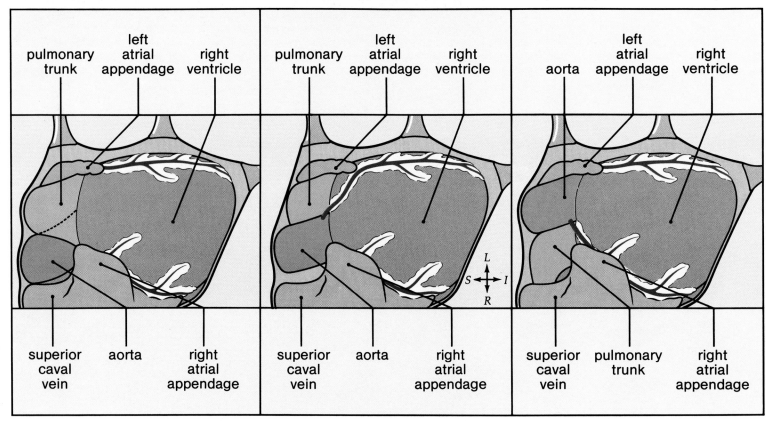

Fig. 7.39 *The three typical arrangements, (left) normal, (middle) anterior and right-sided aorta and (right) anterior and left-sided aorta, found in hearts with double outlet right ventricle with the usual atrial arrangement and atrioventricular concordance, as seen through a median sternotomy.*

Ebstein's malformation is the lesion which most frequently afflicts the left-sided morphologically tricuspid valve. This involves downward displacement of the septal and mural leaflets of the valve (Fig. 7.38), but only rarely is the inlet part of the ventricle dilated and thinned, as occurs so frequently in Ebstein's malformation with atrioventricular concordance. Should valve replacement become necessary, the anterior position of the conduction tissues puts them out of

danger. In this respect it must be mentioned that sometimes there is a normal node and bundle in corrected transposition, either in isolation or as part of a sling. An isolated posterior conduction system is the rule with mirror-image atria (*Wilkinson et al., 1978*) and has been described in a case with the usual atrial arrangement (*Joris & Demoulin, 1981*). In this particular case there was better alignment than usually expected between the inlet and atrial septa. If there

is a posterior node in a patient with Ebstein's anomaly, the conduction system is then at risk.

The other anomaly which affects the left valve, and which can also affect the right (*Becker et al., 1980*), is straddling. This does not alter the origin of the conduction tissues from an anterolateral node but it will markedly increase the risks of surgery (*McGoon et al., 1981*).

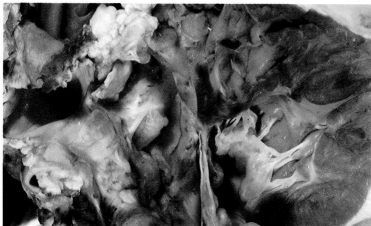

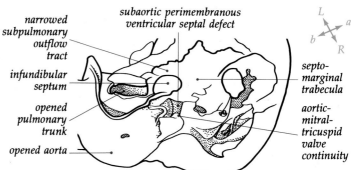

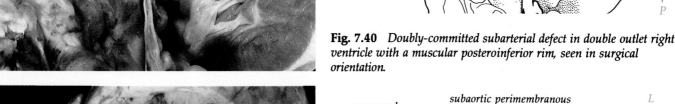

Fig. 7.40 *Doubly-committed subarterial defect in double outlet right ventricle with a muscular posteroinferior rim, seen in surgical orientation.*

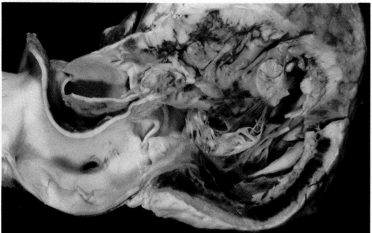

Fig. 7.41 *More or less normally-related great arteries, double outlet right ventricle and a perimembranous subaortic defect, seen in surgical orientation.*

v. Double outlet ventricle

When considering ventriculoarterial connexions we have found it useful to apply the '50 percent law'. Thus, a double outlet ventricle is one which is connected to more than half of both great arteries. In the vast majority of cases there is little question as to the anatomical assignment of an overriding valve, since rarely does it appear to be equally committed to both chambers. It should be emphasized that this assignment is anatomical, for making such designations on the basis of angiography or echocardiography can be misleading. Variations in the angle of view or streaming of the angiographic material can make proper assignment difficult. Nonetheless, if one accepts the '50 percent law' as a pragmatic decision-making approach, the subject of double outlet ventricle becomes straightforward, if not actually simple.

Because a double outlet ventriculo-arterial connexion can exist with such a wide variety of cardiac configurations, the possible combinations seem almost limitless. The cases most frequently encountered are those with both arteries arising from the right ventricle, double outlet right ventricle. Almost invariably a ventricular septal defect is present (*Wilcox et al., 1981*) and it is the interrelationships between the great arteries and the defect that is important to surgeons. Also of obvious significance is the presence of other associated anomalies. Therefore, this section will focus on the relation-

ships of the great arteries as they leave the ventricle (Fig. 7.39), their relationship to the various types of ventricular septal defect and the effect of associated anomalies on surgical considerations. These relationships will be discussed in terms of hearts with the usual atrial arrangement and concordant atrio-ventricular connexions, rather than needlessly complicating an already complex issue by detailing all the rare possibilities that can and do exist. Nevertheless, it should be pointed out that atrial isomerism is often found in these hearts (*De Tommasi et al., 1981*) and in such cases some form of anomalous venous return must be anticipated.

In an analysis of 84 specimens (*Wilkinson, Wilcox & Anderson, 1983*), it was found that in more than half the cases the aortic and pulmonary valves were related more or less 'normally'; in other words, the aortic valve was posterior and to the right of the pulmonary valve, and the pulmonary trunk spiralled round the aorta towards its branching point. In the remainder, the arterial trunks arose from the base of the heart in parallel, as anticipated for complete transposition. For a good proportion of these, the arterial valves were also side by side; otherwise, the aortic valve was anterior. In a few cases the aorta was posteriorly located, usually because the pulmonary trunk was enlarged. In all cases the aorta was to the right. Although none with left-sided aorta were found in this series, such

cases do exist (*Lincoln et al., 1975*).

The anatomy of the ventricular septal defects should be considered in two ways: firstly, with respect to their proximity to the great arteries (*Lev et al., 1972*); and secondly, with respect to their morphology (*Soto et al., 1980*). When combining these two approaches it must be remembered that only the inlet and trabecular muscular components are represented in the interventricular septum. The outlet component is the muscular tissue, if present, between the two 'outlets' in the right ventricle and is exclusively a right ventricular structure. It has been shown that identification of these defects as perimembranous or muscular is extremely helpful in predicting the precise position of the conduction tissue (*Wilcox et al., 1981; Anderson et al., 1983*).

The defect may vary from case to case in relation to the great arteries, but almost invariably the defect can be found cradled between the limbs of the septomarginal trabecula. Its other borders vary depending on several features. The first is whether the septomarginal trabecula fuses with the ventriculoinfundibular fold. If it does, there is a muscular inferior rim to the defect which protects the conduction tissue axis (Fig. 7.40). If it does not, there is arterial-atrioventricular valve continuity and the defect is perimembranous (Fig. 7.41). The second feature is the extent of the ventriculoinfundibular fold.

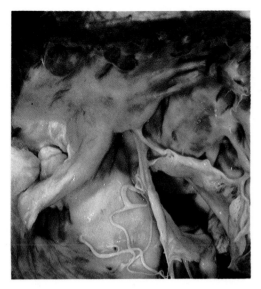

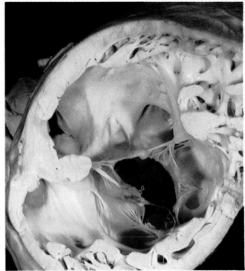

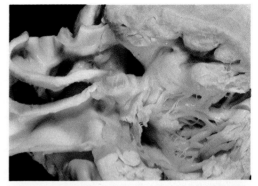

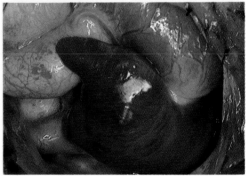

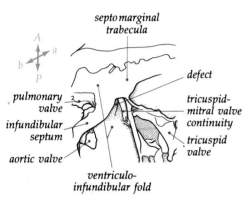

septo marginal trabecula

pulmonary valve

infundibular septum

aortic valve

ventriculo-infundibular fold

defect

tricuspid-mitral valve continuity

tricuspid valve

Fig. 7.42 *Double outlet right ventricle and a perimembranous subaortic defect with an extensive bilateral infundibulum, in surgical orientation.*

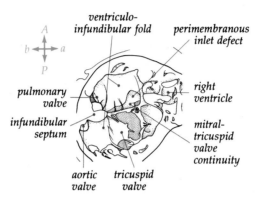

ventriculo-infundibular fold

perimembranous inlet defect

pulmonary valve

infundibular septum

aortic valve

tricuspid valve

right ventricle

mitral-tricuspid valve continuity

Fig. 7.43 *More or less normally-related great arteries and a bilateral infundibulum but with a perimembranous defect in non-committed inlet position, seen in surgical orientation.*

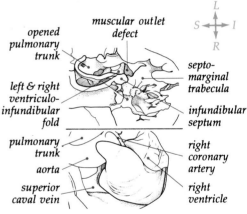

opened pulmonary trunk

muscular outlet defect

left & right ventriculo-infundibular fold

pulmonary trunk

aorta

superior caval vein

septo-marginal trabecula

infundibular septum

right coronary artery

right ventricle

Fig. 7.44 *Double outlet right ventricle: (upper) with subpulmonary ventricular septal defect ('Taussig-Bing malformation'); (lower) operative view of the aorta ascending to the right of and parallel to the pulmonary trunk.*

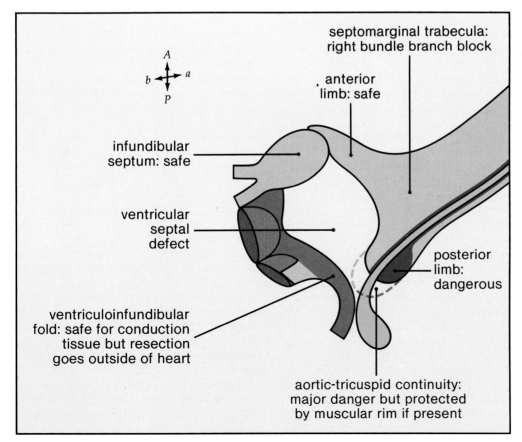

septomarginal trabecula: right bundle branch block

anterior limb: safe

infundibular septum: safe

ventricular septal defect

ventriculoinfundibular fold: safe for conduction tissue but resection goes outside of heart

posterior limb: dangerous

aortic-tricuspid continuity: major danger but protected by muscular rim if present

Fig. 7.45 *Important anatomical information can be gained from the precise identification of the muscular structures which surround the ventricular septal defect in double outlet right ventricle.*

When there is a well formed fold, there is a bilateral infundibulum and the arterial valves are some distance away from the defect (Fig. 7.42). A defect can also be perimembranous because of mitral-tricuspid continuity even when there is a bilateral infundibulum (Fig. 7.43).

The final feature is the relationship of the outlet septum to the other structures. When the outlet septum is attached anteriorly to the trabecular septum, the defect is placed beneath the posterior and right-sided great artery, almost invariably the aorta (Fig. 7.42). When the outlet septum is attached to the ventriculo-infundibular fold or to the posterior limb of the septomarginal trabecula, the defect is placed beneath the left-sided great artery, almost always the pulmonary trunk (Fig. 7.44, upper). When the outlet septum is absent, the defect is doubly-committed (Fig. 7.40).

Thus, if one were to characterize the 'typical' hearts with double outlet right ventricular connexions that might present for operation, two types stand out. The most frequent configuration would be for the aortic valve to be posterior and to the right of the pulmonary artery, associated with a perimembranous subaortic defect (Fig. 7.41). This can be considered a Fallot-like situation. This arterial relationship can also be found with a doubly-committed defect. The second type of heart would have the aorta ascending parallel to the pulmonary trunk, usually either in anterior or side-by-side (Fig. 7.44, lower) position and to the right, with the septal defect being perimembranous or muscular but in subpulmonary position. This is the so-called 'Taussig-Bing' arrangement (Fig. 7.44).

After establishing the above relationships, it is important for the surgeon to identify any other abnormalities in this extremely heterogeneous group of malformations. By far the most common set of anomalies relates to arterial outlet obstruction such as infundibular stenosis, valvular stenosis, coarctation or interrupted aortic arch. The presence of subpulmonary infundibular stenosis is a particularly frequent finding in the Fallot variant (see Chapter 6, v). Coarctation and interrupted arch, together with straddling of the mitral valve, are frequent accompaniments of the 'Taussig-Bing' type (*Parr et al., 1983*). Common atrioventricular valves also occur in a significant number of cases. Unusual coronary artery anatomy is found most frequently when the aorta is in anterior or side-by-side position. In this situation, special consideration is needed when performing a right ventriculotomy.

The importance of careful anatomical analysis in hearts with double outlet right ventricle is underscored by a retrospective analysis of 63 post-mortem specimens concerning possible surgical 'correction' (*Wilcox et al., 1981*). By virtue of the anatomical findings it was concluded that 23 (36 percent) of the hearts could not have been 'corrected'. In another 25 percent the anatomy was judged to be such that very complex, presumably higher risk, procedures would have been required to achieve 'correction'. The remaining 39 percent would have lent themselves to the creation of an intraventricular tunnel of some sort directing left ventricular flow to the aorta. This is the type of procedure done most frequently and most success-fully for this condition (*Kirklin, Harp & McGoon, 1964*).

Surgical and anatomical considerations (Fig. 7.45) for these various procedures relate to the particular combination of

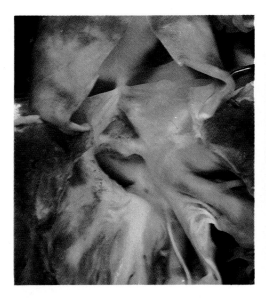
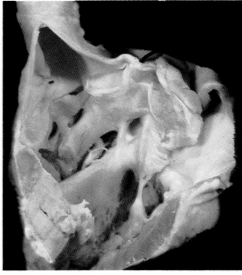

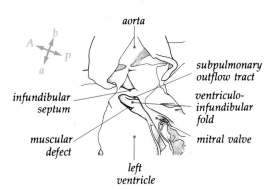

Fig. 7.46 *Left ventricular aspect of double outlet left ventricle, bilateral infundibulum and subaortic defect, in anatomical orientation.*

Fig. 7.47 *Left ventricular aspect of double outlet left ventricle, left-sided anterior aorta and subaortic defect, in anatomical orientation.*

defects. The outlet septum, almost always present, serves as a guide to the arterial valves and their relationships to each other and to the ventricular septal defect. As described above, in cases with subaortic defects the septum usually inserts into the anterior limb of the septomarginal trabecula. With sub-pulmonary defects, it usually inserts into the ventriculoinfundibular fold or into the posterior ventricular septum. This outlet septum is always devoid of any vital structure so it can be resected or used as a secure site for suture anchorage. In contrast, the ventriculoinfundibular fold is not a solid bar of muscle (see Fig. 2.28) and care must be taken to avoid extensive dissection or resection of this structure.

Knowledge of the type of ventricular septal defect will, as in isolated defects (see Chapter 6, ii), give accurate guidance to the disposition of the conduction tissue. Subpulmonary outflow tract obstruction requires the same attention to detail as when dealing with tetralogy of Fallot (see Chapter 6). Other cardiac anomalies will have to be dealt with in the context of the particular cardiac configuration present.

It may not have passed unnoticed that we have discussed this anomaly with little reference to the so-called 'bilateral conus'. This is because we do not believe this

feature to be an integral part of the anomaly. 'Double outlet' describes a connexion and that is what we have defined. The bilateral conus depends simply on whether the ventriculo-infundibular fold separates the atrio-ventricular and arterial valves completely or is attenuated to permit valvar fibrous continuity. Either arrangement can exist with the ventriculoarterial connexion of double outlet ventricle.

Double outlet left ventricle (Figs. 7.46 & 7.47) can present with similar variations in arterial position and relationship to the ventricular septal defect as described for double outlet right ventricle (*Bharati et al., 1978*). Though Otero Coto and co-workers (1983) have pointed out that there have been no published descriptions of the conduction system in double outlet left ventricular connexion, studies from closely related anomalies have been reported (*Anderson, Ho & Becker, 1983; Milo et al., 1980*). These studies imply that the conduction axis is normally disposed when there are otherwise normal segmental connexions. Also, it should be remembered that, as with double outlet right ventricle, double outlet left ventricle can be found with any atrioventricular connexion and the rules for conduction tissue disposition will change accordingly.

7.19

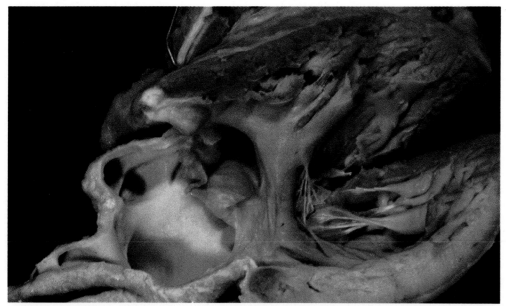

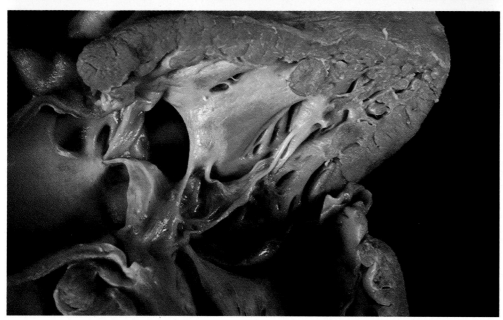

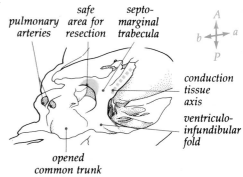

Fig. 7.48 *Opened anterior part of the right ventricle in surgical orientation showing the morphology of a subarterial defect with a muscular posteroinferior rim in a common trunk. The origin of both pulmonary arteries is from the leftward and posterior aspect of the trunk.*

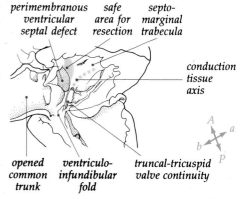

Fig. 7.49 *Common trunk with a perimembranous defect. Compared with Fig. 7.48 the conduction axis is much closer to the posteroinferior margin. The safe area is in a similar position.*

vi. Common arterial trunk

This is defined as a single arterial trunk directly supplying the systemic, pulmonary and coronary arteries. In this way the anomaly is distinguished from the other types of single outlet ventriculo-arterial connexion, namely a solitary aortic trunk with pulmonary atresia or a solitary pulmonary trunk with aortic atresia. Either of these arrangements is appropriately described as single outlet when it is not possible to determine the ventricular origin of the atretic great artery. For the purposes of definition, it is also our convention to describe a common trunk only when it is guarded by a common arterial valve (*Crupi, Macartney & Anderson, 1977*). In this we are following the usual practice, although some authorities (*Van Praagh & Van Praagh, 1965; Calder et al., 1976*) have suggested that common trunks can have two discrete outflow tracts and separate aortic and pulmonary valves. We believe that from a surgical viewpoint it is better to consider the latter lesions as large aortopulmonary windows. They pose far

less severe problems for repair than those malformations with a common outflow tract which are discussed here.

It is also worthwhile to consider one further anomaly before leaving the vexatious realm of definitions: the lesion characterized by having a solitary arterial trunk with no evidence whatsoever of intrapericardial pulmonary arteries. The controversy as to whether the solitary great vessel is a common trunk ('truncus type IV') or an aorta is readily resolved by describing it as a solitary arterial trunk (*Thiene & Anderson, 1983*). From the surgical viewpoint, the treatment is more akin to that for pulmonary atresia (see Chapter 6) than for common arterial trunks.

The anatomical features of a common trunk which determine the success of surgical treatment are its connexion to the ventricular mass, the state of the truncal valve, the morphology of the ventricular septal defect and the arrangement of the great arteries. Although common trunks can exist with any atrioventricular connexion, it is very rarely found with other

than atrioventricular concordance. The trunk usually overrides the ventricular septum and is connected more or less equally to the right and left ventricles. The septal defect is present because of the complete lack of the infundibular septum and thus it is directly subarterial. Usually it is cradled between the limbs of the septomarginal trabecula, with the posterior limb fusing with the ventriculo-infundibular fold (Fig. 7.48). As with other defects of this type (see Chapter 6), the muscle bundle thus formed serves to buttress the conduction tissue axis away from the septal crest. More rarely, there can be truncal-tricuspid continuity, which puts the conduction axis much more at risk during closure when connecting the common trunk to the left ventricle (Fig. 7.49). In the rare instance that the defect is restrictive, it is usually because the common trunk is connected solely or mostly to the right ventricle, often with a subtruncal infundibulum (Fig. 7.50). If necessary the defect may be enlarged along its anterosuperior margins.

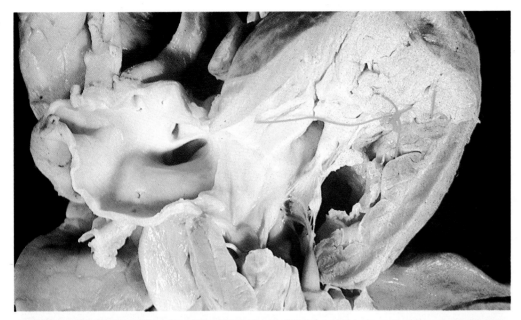

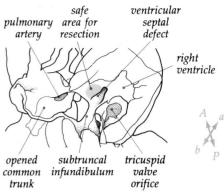

Fig. 7.50 *Common trunk opened as in Figs. 7.48 & 7.49. The trunk arises exclusively from the right ventricle and has a subtruncal infundibulum. The defect is restrictive and the safe area for resection is superimposed.*

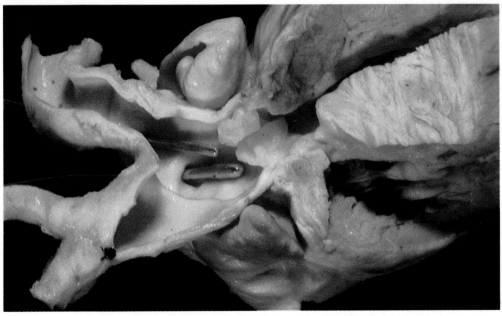

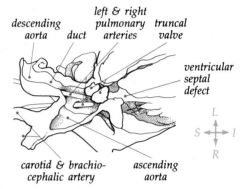

Fig. 7.51 *Section at right angles to the septum in a common trunk with interrupted arch, in surgical orientation. The truncal valve is connected mostly to the left ventricle and the blood supply to the lower body is duct-dependent.*

After surgical repair of a common trunk following the Rastelli technique (*Rastelli, Titus & McGoon, 1967*), the truncal valve effectively becomes the aortic valve. Valvar incompetence or stenosis, if present, is therefore of considerable significance. Although dysplastic truncal valves have been encountered with some frequency in autopsy studies of infant hearts (*Becker, Becker & Edwards, 1971*), they do not seem to pose a major problem in surgical repair in infancy. The common trunk may also be predominantly connected to the left ventricle, but this variation works in the surgeon's favour and does not pose additional problems.

Variation in great arterial morphology is found in both the pulmonary and aortic pathways. Following the classical studies of Collett and Edwards (1949), a common trunk is usually classified according to the mode of pulmonary arterial origin. The most common patterns are either for the two pulmonary arteries to arise from a short confluent channel ('type I') or for the arteries to arise

separately and directly from the left posterior aspect of the trunk ('type II'). Presence of a short pulmonary confluence would certainly facilitate banding, but this procedure is now performed with far less frequency in specialized centres. Either of these two patterns permits easy connexion to a right ventricular conduit during complete repair. The much rarer variant, in which each pulmonary artery arises from the side of the trunk ('type III') makes complete repair more difficult though not impossible. As described above, we believe that the so-called 'truncus type IV', where there is no evidence of intrapericardial pulmonary arteries, is best described as a solitary arterial trunk. The possibility of successful surgical treatment is dictated by the pattern of pulmonary arterial supply via the major aortopulmonary collateral arteries.

Categorization of common trunks tends to concentrate on the pulmonary arteries, but it is the pattern of the aortic arch which is of much more significance surgically. Usually the aorta arises in its

anticipated position or, more rarely, anteriorly (*Angelini et al., 1977*), but continues to supply the head, neck and arm arteries and the descending aorta. The variant in which the aortic arch is interrupted is the pattern which will create problems for the surgeon. In this arrangement the ascending aorta supplies all or only part of the head, neck and arm arteries (*Calder et al., 1976*). Usually the interruption is at the isthmus but it can occur proximal to the origin of the left subclavian artery. In either case, the descending aorta is supplied by the duct (Fig. 7.51). It is therefore imperative to recognize this arrangement and make appropriate modifications if surgical repair is contemplated (*Gomes & McGoon, 1971*). Common trunks with interruption are not infrequent, being found in up to one-fifth of autopsy series (*Van Praagh & Van Praagh, 1965; Bharati et al., 1974; Calder et al., 1976; Crupi et al., 1977*). Other rare variations in arterial pattern occur in association with common trunks, such as crossed pulmonary arteries (*Becker, Becker & Edwards, 1970*).

Anderson, R.H., Becker, A.E., Arnold, R. & Wilkinson, J.L. (1974) The conducting tissues in congenitally corrected transposition. *Circulation*, **50,** 911–923.

Anderson, R.H., Becker, A.E. & Gerlis, L.M. (1975) The pulmonary outflow tract in classically corrected transposition. *Journal of Thoracic and Cardiovascular Surgery*, **69,** 747–757.

Anderson, R.H., Becker, A.E., Wilcox, B.R., Macartney, F.J. & Wilkinson, J.L. (1983) Surgical anatomy of double outlet right ventricle – a reappraisal. *American Journal of Cardiology*, **52,** 555–559.

Anderson, R.H., Danielson, G.K., Maloney, J.D. & Becker, A.E. (1978) Atrioventricular bundle in corrected transposition. *Annals of Thoracic Surgery*, **26,** 95–96.

Anderson, R.H., Ho, S.Y. & Becker, A.E. (1983) The surgical anatomy of the conduction tissues. *Thorax*, **38,** 408–420.

Anderson, R.H., Tynan, M.J., Freedom, R.M., Quero-Jimenez, M., Macartney, F.J., Shinebourne, E.A., Wilkinson, J.L. & Becker, A.E. (1979) Ventricular morphology in the univentricular heart. *Herz*, **4,** 184–197.

Angelini, P., Verdugo, A.L., Illera, J.P. & Leachman, R.D. (1977) Truncus arteriosus communis. Unusual case associated with transposition. *Circulation*, **56,** 1107–1110.

Arteaga, M.M., Fernandez-Espino, R., Quero-Jimenez, M., Noriega, N. & de la Cruz, M.V. (1981) Discordancia ventriculo-arterial con aorta posterior. Estudio anatomico de nueve casos. *Revista Espanola de Cardiologia*, **2,** 277–287.

Aubert, J., Pannatier, A., Couvelly, J.P., Unal, D., Rouault, F. & Delarue. A. (1978) Transposition of the great arteries. New technique for anatomical correction: case report. *British Heart Journal*, **40,** 204-208.

Becker, A.E., Becker, M.J. & Edwards, J.E. (1971) Pathology of the semi-lunar valve in persistent truncus arteriosus. *Journal of Thoracic and Cardiovascular Surgery*, **62,** 16–26.

Becker, A.E., Becker, M.J. & Edwards, J.E. (1970) Anomalies associated with coarctation of the aorta. Particular reference to infancy. *Circulation*, **41,** 1067–1075.

Becker, A.E., Ho, S.Y., Caruso, G., Milo, S. & Anderson, R.H. (1980) Straddling right atrioventricular valves in atrio-ventricular discordance. *Circulation*, **61,** 1133–1141.

Bharati, S., Lev, M., Stewart, R., McAllister, H.A.Jr. & Kirklin, J.W. (1978) The morphologic spectrum of double outlet left ventricle and its surgical significance. *Circulation*, **58,** 558–565.

Bharati, S., McAllister, H.A.Jr., Rosenquist, G.C., Miller, R.A., Tatooles, C.J. & Lev, M. (1974) The surgical anatomy of truncus arteriosus communis. *Journal of Thoracic and Cardiovascular Surgery*, **67,** 501–510.

Buchler, J.R., Bembom, J.C. & Buchler, R.D. (1984) Transposition of the great arteries with posterior aorta and subaortic conus: anatomical and surgical correlation. *International Journal of Cardiology*, **5,** 13–18.

Calder, L., Van Praagh, R., Van Praagh, S., Sears, W.P., Corwin, R., Levy, A., Keith, J.D. & Paul, M.H. (1976) Truncus arteriosus communis. Clinical, angiographic, and pathologic findings in 100 patients. *American Heart Journal*, **92,** 23–38.

Collett, R.W. & Edwards, J.E. (1949) Persistent truncus arteriosus. A classification according to anatomic types. *Surgical Clinics of North America*, **29,** 1245–1270.

Crupi, G., Macartney, F.J. & Anderson, R.H. (1977) Persistent truncus arteriosus. A study of 66 autopsy cases with special reference to definition and morphogenesis. *American Journal of Cardiology*, **40,** 569-578.

Damus, P.S., Thomson, N.B.Jr. & McLoughlin, T.G. (1982) Arterial repair without coronary relocation for complete transposition of the great vessels with ventricular septal defect: report of case. *Journal of Thoracic and Cardiovascular Surgery*, **83,** 316–318.

Danielson, G.K., McGoon, D.C., Maloney, J.D. & Ritter, D.G. (1978) Surgery of primitive ventricle with outlet chamber. In *Paediatric Cardiology 1977*, pp. 381-387. Edited by R.H. Anderson & E.A. Shinebourne. Edinburgh: Churchill Livingstone.

De Leval, M., Bastos, P., Stark, J., Taylor, J.F.N., Macartney, F.J. & Anderson, R.H. (1979) Surgical technique to reduce the risks of heart block following closure of ventricular septal defect in atrioventricular discordance. *Journal of Thoracic and Cardiovascular Surgery*, **78,** 515–526.

De Tommasi, S.M., Daliento, L., Ho, S.Y., Macartney, F.J. & Anderson, R.H. (1981) Analysis of atrioventricular junction, ventricular mass and ventriculoarterial junction in 43 specimens with atrial isomerism. *British Heart Journal*, **45,** 236–247.

Doty, D.B. & Knott, H.W. (1977) Hypoplastic left heart syndrome. Experience with an operation to establish functionally normal circulation. *Journal of Thoracic and Cardiovascular Surgery*, **74,** 624-630.

Doty, D.B., Marvin, W.J.Jr. & Lauer, R.M. (1981) Modified Fontan procedure. Methods to achieve direct anastomosis of right atrium to pulmonary artery. *Journal of Thoracic and Cardiovascular Surgery*, **81,** 470–475.

Doty, D.B., Truesdell, S.C. & Marvin, W.J.Jr. (1983) Techniques to avoid injury of the conduction tissue during the surgical treatment of corrected transposition. *Circulation*, **68 II,** 63–69.

Essed, C.E., Ho, S.Y., Hunter, S. & Anderson R.H. (1980) Atrioventricular conduction system in univentricular heart of right ventricular type with right-sided rudimentary chamber. *Thorax*, **35,** 123–127.

Fontan, F., Choussat, A., Brom, A.G., Chauve, A., Deville, C. & Casto-Cels, A. (1978) Repair of tricuspid atresia – surgical considerations and results. In *Paediatric Cardiology 1977*, pp 567–580. Edited by R.H. Anderson & E.A. Shinebourne. Edinburgh: Churchill Livingstone.

Freedom, R.M., Sondheimer, H., Dische, R. & Rowe, R.D. (1977) Development of 'subaortic stenosis' after pulmonary arterial banding for common ventricle. *American Journal of Cardiology*, **39,** 78–83.

Gale, A.W., Danielson, G.K., McGoon, D.C. & Mair, D.D. (1979) Modified Fontan operation for univentricular heart and complicated congenital lesions. *Journal of Thoracic and Cardiovascular Surgery*, **78,** 831–838.

Girod, D.A., Lima, R.C., Anderson, R.H., Ho, S.Y., Rigby, M.L. & Quaegebeur, J.M. (1984) Double inlet ventricle: morphological analysis and surgical implications in 32 cases. *Journal of Thoracic and Cardiovascular Surgery*. In press.

Gittenberger-de Groot, A.C., Sauer, U., Oppenheimer-Dekker, A. & Quaegebeur, J. (1983) Coronary arterial anatomy in transposition of the great arteries: a morphologic study. In *Pediatric Cardiology Supplement 1*, **4,** 15–24.

Gomes, M.M.R. & McGoon, D.C. (1971) Truncus arteriosus with interruption of the aortic arch: report of a case successfully repaired. *Mayo Clinic Proceedings*, **46,** 40–43.

Hamilton, D.I., Arnold, R. & Wilkinson, J.L. (1978) Surgery of the univentricular heart without outlet chamber. In *Paediatric Cardiology 1977*, pp 388–395. Edited by R.H. Anderson & E.A. Shinebourne. Edinburgh: Churchill Livingstone.

Henry, J.N., Devloo, R.A.E., Ritter, D.G., Mair, D.D., Davis, G.D. & Danielson, G.K. (1974) Tricuspid atresia. Surgical 'correction' in two patients using porcine xenograft valves. *Mayo Clinic Proceedings*, **49,** 803–810.

Isaacson, R., Titus, J.L., Meridith, J., Feldt, R.H. & McGoon, D.C. (1972) Apparent interruption of atrial conduction pathways after surgical repair of transposition of the great arteries. *American Journal of Cardiology*, **30,** 533–535.

Jatene, A.D., Fontes, V.F., Paulista, P.P., De Souza, L.C.B., Neger, F., Galantier, M. & Souza, J.E.M.R. (1976) Anatomic correction of transposition of the great vessels. *Journal of Thoracic and Cardiovascular Surgery*, **72,** 364–370.

Joris, H. & Demoulin, J.C. (1981) Corrected transposition of the great arteries in adults. One case report and a review of the literature on the evolution and anatomical study with histology of the conduction system. *Archives des Maladies du Coeur et des Vaisseaux*, **74,** 951–960.

Kaye, M.P. (1975) Anatomic correction of transposition of great arteries. *Mayo Clinic Proceedings*, **50,** 638–640.

Kirklin, J.W., Harp, R.A. & McGoon, D.C. (196) Surgical treatment of origin of both vessels from right ventricle, including cases of pulmonary stenosis. *Journal of Thoracic and Cardiovascular Surgery*, **48,** 1026–1036.

Kupersmith, J., Krongrad, E., Gersony, W.M. & Bowman, F.O. (1974) Electrophysiologic identification of the specialized conduction system in corrected transposition of the great arteries. *Circulation*, **50,** 795–800.

Lev, M., Bharati, S., Meng, C.C.L., Liberthson, R.R., Paul, M.H. & Idriss, F. (1972) A concept of double-outlet right ventricle. *Journal of Thoracic and Cardiovascular Surgery*, **64,** 271–281.

Lincoln, C.R., Anderson, R.H., Shinebourne, E.A., English, T.A.H. & Wilkinson, J.L. (1975) Double outlet right ventricle with l-malposition of the aorta. *British Heart Journal*, **37,** 453-463.

Lincoln, C.R., Hasse, J., Anderson, R.H. & Shinebourne, E.A. (1976) Surgical correction in complete levotransposition of the great arteries with an unusual subaortic ventricular septal defect. *American Journal of Cardiology*, **38,** 344–351.

Losekoot, T.G., Anderson, R.H., Becker, A.E., Danielson, G.K. & Soto, B. (1983) Anatomy and embryology. In: *Congenitally Corrected Transposition*, pp 21–41. Edinburgh: Churchill Livingstone.

McGoon, D.C., Danielson, G.K., Ritter, D.G., Wallace, R.B., Maloney, J.D. & Marcelletti, C. (1977) Correction of the univentricular heart having two atrioventricular valves. *Journal of Thoracic and Cardiovascular Surgery*, **74,** 218–226.

McGoon, D.C., Danielson, G.K., Wallace, R.B. & Puga, F.J. (1981) Surgical implications of straddling atrioventricular valves. In *Paediatric Cardiology Volume 3*, pp 431–440. Edited by A.E. Becker, T.G. Losekoot, C. Marcelletti & R.H. Anderson. Edinburgh: Churchill Livingstone.

McKay, R., Pacifico, A.D., Blackstone, E.H., Kirklin, J.W., & Bargeron, L.M.Jr. (1982) Septation of the univentricular heart with left subaortic outlet chamber. *Journal of Thoracic and Cardiovascular Surgery*, **84,** 77–87.

Mickell, J.J., Mathews, R.A., Park, S.C., Lenox, C.C., Fricker, F.J., Neches, W.H. & Zuberbuhler, J.R. (1980) Left atrioventricular valve atresia: clinical management. *Circulation*, **61,** 123–127.

Milo, S., Ho, S.Y., Wilkinson, J.L. & Anderson, R.H. (1980) The surgical anatomy and atrioventricular conduction tissues of hearts with isolated ventricular septal defects. *Journal of Thoracic and Cardiovascular Surgery*, **79,** 244–255.

Norwood, W.I., Kirklin, J.W. & Sanders, S.P. (1980) Hypoplastic left heart syndrome: experience with palliative surgery. *American Journal of Cardiology*, **45,** 87–91.

Norwood, W.I., Lang, P. & Hansen, D.D. (1983) Physiologic repair of the aortic atresia-hypoplastic left heart syndrome. *New England Journal of Medicine*, **308,** 23–26.

Okamura, J. & Konno, S. (1973) Two types of ventricular septal defect in corrected transposition of the great arteries. Reference to surgical approaches. *American Heart Journal*, **85,** 483–490.

Otero Coto, E., Quero-Jimenez, M., Anderson, R.H., Castenada, A.R., Freedom, R.M., Attie, F., Kreutzer, E., Kreutzer, G. & Becker, A.E. (1983) Double outlet left ventricle. In *Paediatric Cardiology Volume 5*, pp 451–465. Edited by R.H. Anderson, F.J. Macartney, E.A. Shinebourne & M.J. Tynan. Edinburgh: Churchill Livingstone.

Pacifico, A.D., McKay, R., Kirklin, J.W. & Kirklin, J.K. (1983) Surgical management of the univentricular heart. In *Paediatric Cardiology Volume 5*, pp 276–292. Edited by R.H. Anderson, F.J. Macartney, E.A. Shinebourne & M.J. Tynan.

Parr, G.V.S., Waldhausen, J.A., Bharati, S., Lev, M., Fripp, R. & Whitman, V. (1983) Coarctation in Taussig-Bing malformation of the heart. Surgical signficiance. *Journal of Thoracic and Cardiovascular Surgery*, **86,** 280–287.

Rastelli, G.C., Titus, J.L., & McGoon, D.C. (1967) Homograft of ascending aorta as a right ventricular outflow: an experimental approach to the repair of truncus arteriosus. *Archives of Surgery*, **95,** 698–708.

Rowlatt, U.F. (1962) Coronary artery distribution in complete transposition. *Journal of American Medical Association*, **179,** 269–278.

Scalia, D., Russo, P., Anderson, R.H., Macartney, F.J., Hegerty, A.S., Ho, S.Y., Daliento, L. & Thiene, G. (1984) The surgical anatomy of hearts with no direct communication between the right atrium and the ventricular mass – so-called tricuspid atresia. *Journal of Thoracic and Cardiovascular Surgery*, **87,** 743–755.

Shaher, R.M. & Puddu, G.C. (1966) Coronary arterial anatomy in complete transposition of the great arteries. *American Journal of Cardiology*, **17,** 355–361.

Shore, D., Jones, O., Rigby, M.L., Anderson, R.H. & Lincoln, C.R. (1982) Atresia of left atrioventricular connection. Surgical considerations. *British Heart Journal*, **47,** 35–40.

Soto, B., Becker, A.E., Moulaert, A.J., Lie, J.T., & Anderson, R.H. (1980) Classification of ventricular septal defects. *British Heart Journal*, **43,** 332–343.

Southall, D.P., Keeton, B.R., Leanage, R., Lam, L., Joseph, M.C., Anderson, R.H., Lincoln, C.R. & Shinebourne, E.A. (1980) Cardiac rhythm and conduction before and after Mustard's operation for complete transposition of the great arteries. *British Heart Journal*, **43,** 21–30.

Stansel, H.G. (1975) A new operation for d-loop transposition of the great vessels. *Annals of Thoracic Surgery*, **19,** 565–567.

Stefanelli, G., Kirklin, J.W., Naftal, D.C., Blackstone, E.H., Pacifico, A.D., Kirklin, J.K., Soto, B. & Bargeron, L.M. (1984) Early and intermediate-term (10 year) results of surgery for univentricular atrioventricular connexion (single ventricle). *American Journal of Cardiology*, **88,** 590–602.

Stewart, S., Manning, J. & Siegel, L. (1977) Automated identification of cardiac conduction tissue in L-TGV and Ebstein's anomaly. *Annals of Thoracic Surgery*, **23,** 215–220.

Thiene, G. & Anderson, R.H. (1983) Pulmonary atresia with ventricular septal defect. In *Paediatric Cardiology Volume 5*, pp 80–101. Edited by R.H. Anderson, F.J. Macartney, E.A. Shinebourne & M.J. Tynan. Edinburgh: Churchill Livingstone.

Tynan, M.J. & Anderson, R.H. (1979) Terminology of transposition of the great arteries. In *Paediatric Cardiology Volume 2, Heart Disease in the Newborn*, pp 341–349. Edited by M.J. Godman & R.M. Marquis. Edinburgh: Churchill Livingstone.

Ullal, R.R., Anderson, R.H. & Lincoln, C.R. (1979) Mustard's operation modified to avoid dysrhythmias and pulmonary and systemic venous obstruction. *Journal of Thoracic and Cardiovascular Surgery*, **78,** 431–439.

Van Mierop, L.H.S. (1971) Transposition of the great arteries. Clarification or further confusion? Editorial. *American Journal of Cardiology*, **28,** 735–738.

Van Praagh, R., Perez-Trevino, C., Lopez-Cuellar, M., Baker, F.W., Zuberbuhler, J.R., Quero, M., Perez, V.M., Moreno, F. & Van Praagh, S. (1971) Transposition of the great arteries with posterior aorta, anterior pulmonary artery, subpulmonary conus and fibrous continuity between aortic and atrioventricular valves. *American Journal of Cardiology*, **28,** 621–631.

Van Praagh, R. & Van Praagh, S. (1965) The anatomy of common aortico-pulmonary trunk (truncus arteriosus communis) and its embryologic implications. *American Journal of Cardiology*, **16,** 406–426.

Wilcox, B.R., Henry, G.W. & Anderson, R.H. (1983) The transmitral approach to left ventricular outflow tract obstruction. *Annals of Thoracic Surgery*, **35,** 288–293.

Wilcox, B.R., Ho, S.Y., Macartney, F.J., Becker, A.E., Gerlis, L.M. & Anderson, R.H. (1981) Surgical anatomy of double-outlet right ventricle with situs solitus and atrioventricular concordance. *Journal of Thoracic and Cardiovascular Surgery*, **82,** 405–417.

Wilkinson, J.L., Anderson, R.H., Arnold, R., Hamilton, D.I. & Smith, A. (1976) The conducting tissues in primitive ventricular hearts without an outlet chamber. *Circulation*, **53,** 930–938.

Wilkinson, J.L., Arnold, R., Anderson, R.H. & Acerete, F. (1975) 'Posterior' transposition reconsidered. *British Heart Journal*, **37,** 757–766.

Wilkinson, J.L., Smith, A., Lincoln, C.R. & Anderson, R.H. (1978) The conducting tissues in congenitally corrected transposition with situs inversus. *British Heart Journal*, **40,** 41–48.

Wilkinson, J.L., Wilcox, B.R. & Anderson, R.H. (1983) Double outlet ventricle. In *Paediatric Cardiology Volume 5*, pp 397–407. Edited by R.H. Anderson, F.J. Macartney, E.A. Shinebourne & M.J. Tynan. Edinburgh: Churchill Livingstone.

Yacoub, M.H. & Radley-Smith, R. (1978) Anatomy of the coronary arteries in transposition of the great arteries and methods for their transfer in anatomical correction. *Thorax*, **33,** 418–424.

8 Abnormalities of the Great Vessels

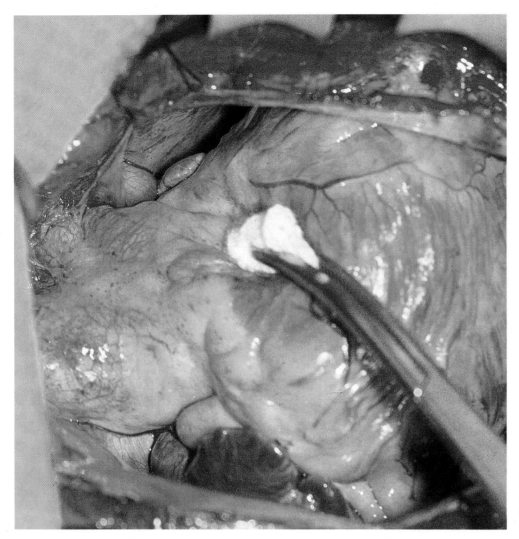

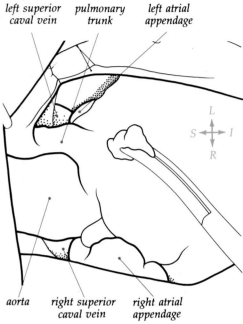

left superior caval vein   pulmonary trunk   left atrial appendage

aorta   right superior caval vein   right atrial appendage

Fig. 8.1 *Operative view through a median sternotomy of a left superior caval vein entering the pericardial cavity between the left atrial appendage and the pulmonary trunk.*

i. Anomalous systemic venous drainage

Abnormal systemic venous connexions are usually of little surgical significance since their clinical consequences are limited. These anomalies are apt to be encountered as the surgeon pursues a more complex associated intracardiac anomaly. They may be grouped into the following categories: absence or abnormal drainage of the right caval vein(s); persistence or abnormal drainage of the left caval vein(s); and abnormal hepatic connexions. Abnormalities of the coronary sinus usually fall into one of these groups, except the 'unroofed' coronary sinus which was discussed in Chapter 6, i.

Abnormalities of the right superior caval vein are extremely rare. It may be diminished in size or it may be completely absent when the venous return from the head, neck and arms passes through a persistent left superior caval vein to the right atrium by way of the coronary sinus or, rarely, directly into the left atrium. Only this last situation requires surgical intervention. The other conditions, if encountered during an open-heart operation, would require some adjustment from the usual cannulation technique. Though there is no definite evidence to this effect, we would not expect these abnormalities to

affect the location of the sinus node.

The right inferior caval vein can be absent at its cavoatrial junction or be in the abdomen with its venous return being directed to the right atrium through the azygos or hemiazygos system. The azygos return can be to the left-sided atrium, producing right-to-left shunting. (Right-to-left shunting can also be an iatrogenic phenomenon occasionally observed when low-lying atrial septal defects are improperly closed; see Chapter 6, i.) Such azygos return is seen most frequently with left atrial isomerism when the hepatic veins drain independently into the right or left atrium. It can also occur in individuals with lateralized atria, and the hepatic veins then connect to the right atrium through a suprahepatic segment of the inferior caval vein.

A persistent left superior caval vein is joined to the right superior caval vein by an innominate vein in about sixty percent of reported cases (*Winter, 1954*). In this arrangement, the left caval vein can simply be clamped or ligated to avoid flooding the field when the heart is opened. If connexions with the right vein are not apparent, a trial period of occlusion will usually indicate whether there will be problems with venous hypertension. Not infrequently, a left superior caval vein is found in patients with cyanotic heart disease, it being

reported in as many as twenty percent of patients with tetralogy of Fallot and eight percent of patients with Eisenmenger's syndrome (*Bankl, 1977*). This venous channel can be the route of partial anomalous pulmonary venous connexion or it can empty through the left-sided pulmonary veins into the left atrium. It can also empty directly into the left atrium ('unroofed' coronary sinus). Much more frequently it is encountered as an isolated lesion which usually receives the hemiazygos vein before penetrating the pericardium and passing between the left atrial appendage and the left pulmonary veins (Figs. 8.1). It then connects with the coronary sinus behind the heart to empty into the right atrium through a larger than normal orifice. In such hearts the Thebesian valve is often attenuated or absent.

Though relatively rare, there may be a persistent left inferior caval vein (*Anderson et al., 1955*) which may drain by way of the azygos system to the superior caval vein. As discussed above, this 'azygos continuation' of the inferior caval vein is commonly found with left atrial isomerism (*Moller et al., 1967*). Exceedingly rarely the inferior caval vein may drain directly into the left atrium (*Venables, 1963*).

Another anomaly which, although rare, warrants consideration is the levoatrial

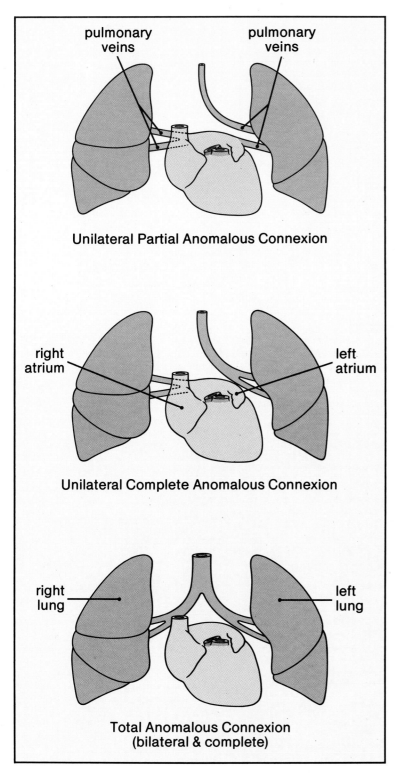

Unilateral Partial Anomalous Connexion

Unilateral Complete Anomalous Connexion

Total Anomalous Connexion
(bilateral & complete)

Fig. 8.2 *Unilateral complete or partial anomalous connexion of the pulmonary veins. Bilateral complete anomalous connexion produces total anomalous drainage.*

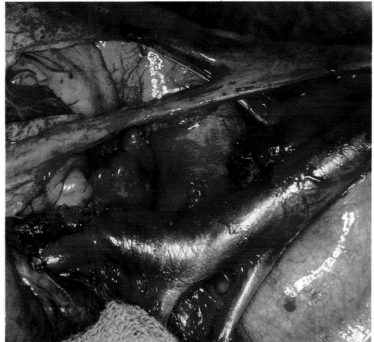

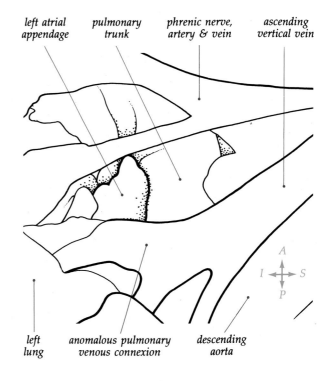

Fig. 8.3 *Operative view through a left lateral thoracotomy of unilateral complete anomalous connexion of the left pulmonary veins to an ascending vertical vein.*

cardinal vein (*Edwards & DuShane, 1950*). This is a channel which connects the left atrium to the systemic venous system and is invariably found with associated lesions such as mitral atresia, where it functions as the only route for pulmonary venous return. Then, although the pulmonary veins are normally connected to the morphologically left atrium, the pattern of venous return is comparable to the 'snowman' type of anomalous pulmonary venous return (see below).

ii. Anomalous pulmonary venous drainage

Very rarely the pulmonary veins may be obstructed or totally atretic at their atrial junction (*Lucas et al., 1962; Mortensson & Lundstrom, 1974*). Much more commonly, abnormalities of the pulmonary venous system take the form of anomalous connexion. Because of the plethora of possibilities for abnormal pulmonary venous connexions (*Nakib et al., 1967; Bharati & Lev, 1973; DeLisle et al., 1976*), it is particularly important that they be

described as specifically and as unambiguously as possible (Fig. 8.2). The pulmonary veins connect anomalously when they are not joined to the morphologically left atrium. Consequently, if all the veins from one lung connect to a site other than the left atrium, the arrangement can be described as complete unilateral anomalous pulmonary venous connexion (Fig. 8.3). If all the veins from both lungs connect to sites other than the morphologically left atrium, there is total anomalous

8.3

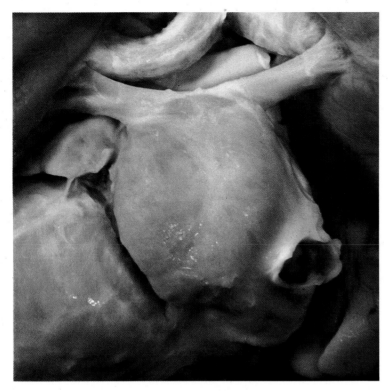

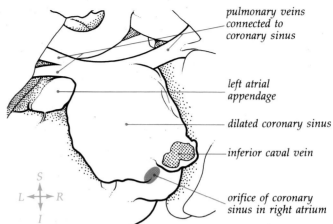

pulmonary veins connected to coronary sinus

left atrial appendage

dilated coronary sinus

inferior caval vein

orifice of coronary sinus in right atrium

Fig. 8.4 *Anatomically orientated posterior view of total anomalous pulmonary venous connexion to the coronary sinus. The sinus is grossly dilated because surgical correction several months previously had produced stenosis in the newly constructed pathway to the left atrium (see Fig. 8.7).*

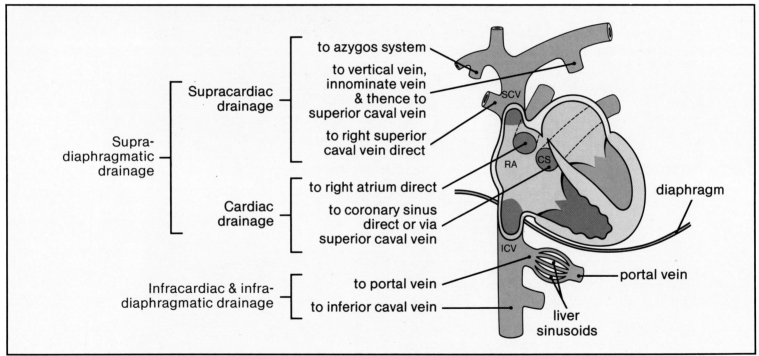

Supra-diaphragmatic drainage

Supracardiac drainage
- to azygos system
- to vertical vein, innominate vein & thence to superior caval vein
- to right superior caval vein direct

Cardiac drainage
- to right atrium direct
- to coronary sinus direct or via superior caval vein

Infracardiac & infra-diaphragmatic drainage
- to portal vein
- to inferior caval vein

diaphragm

portal vein

liver sinusoids

Fig. 8.5 *Sites of anomalous pulmonary venous connexion and their categorization. The pulmonary venous channels are not illustrated.*

pulmonary venous connexion (Fig. 8.4). This, of necessity, implies bilateral complete anomalous connexion.

Any combination can be readily described by treating each lung as an entity (unilateral, partial or complete anomalous connexion; Fig. 8.2). The unifying lesion in all of these combinations is the connexion of one or more pulmonary veins to the systemic venous system or to the right atrium (Fig. 8.5). It is therefore equally important that the site of drainage be identified. Historically, these have been described as supradiaphragmatic or infradiaphragmatic. The supradiaphragmatic group can be subdivided into supracardiac (Fig. 8.6,

upper) and cardiac groups. Supracardiac drainage may be to a right or left superior caval vein, the innominate vein or even the azygos vein. Connexion to the innominate vein is most frequent and the combination of vertical vein and innominate vein (Fig. 8.6, lower) draining to the superior caval vein produces the typical 'snowman' configuration seen on chest radiography. Cardiac drainage enters the right atrium directly or through the coronary sinus (Fig. 8.4). Infra-diaphragmatic drainage is usually total except when there is partial right-sided drainage into the inferior caval vein. This produces the 'scimitar syndrome', a name taken from its roentgenographic

appearance (*Neill et al., 1960*). In the usual infradiaphragmatic connexion, the common channel connecting both lungs lies outside the pericardium posterior to the left atrium. A vertical vein drains through the diaphragm as a single channel to enter the inferior caval vein, the portal vein or the venous duct.

The salient anatomical features relating to surgical repair of anomalous pulmonary connexions include the type of abnormal connexion (for example, total, unilateral or mixed), the site of drainage, and the proximity of the anomalous veins to the left atrium. As pointed out in Chapter 6, i, a superior sinus venosus atrial septal defect is often

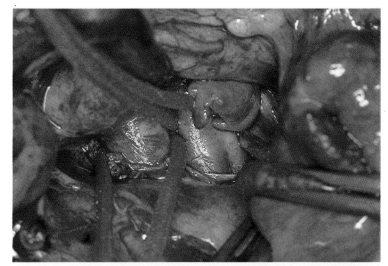

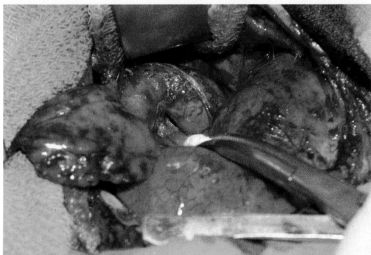

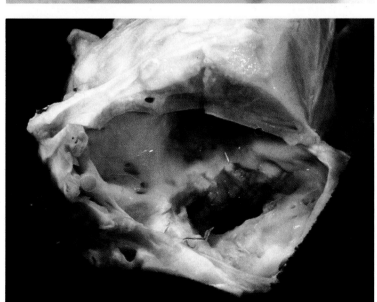

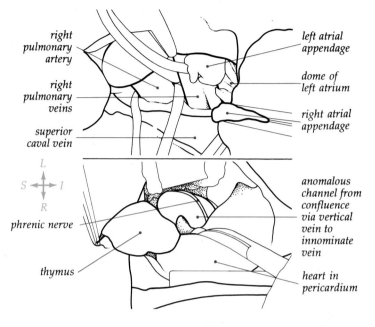

Fig. 8.6 *Total anomalous pulmonary venous return: (upper) operative view through a median sternotomy. The pulmonary veins from the right lung are retropericardial, lying between the right pulmonary artery and dome of the left atrium; (lower) the vertical vein joins the confluence of pulmonary veins to the innominate vein.*

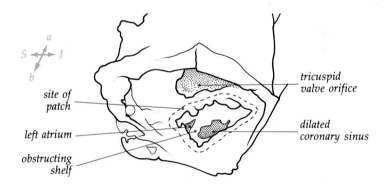

Fig. 8.7 *The heart in Fig. 8.4 was corrected by cutting the coronary sinus back into the coexisting oval fossa defect and placing a patch (here removed) across the orifice of the sinus and the oval fossa defect. Unfortunately, the wall between the enlarged sinus and left atrium was not removed sufficiently ('unroofing' the sinus), thus producing an obstructive shelf.*

accompanied by anomalous drainage of the right pulmonary veins to the superior caval vein. The need to safeguard the sinus node and its blood supply has already been emphasized.

Other sites of drainage or potential sites of anastomosis often require an extensive atrial anastomosis to guard against pulmonary venous obstruction post-operatively. The appropriate landmarks must be borne in mind. Two types of anomalous connexion pose particular problems. The first is when the

anomalous venous return is by way of the coronary sinus (Fig. 8.4) with a common 'party wall' between the coronary sinus and the left atrium. The logical repair is to incise this wall to unroof the sinus. At the same time, the orifice of the coronary sinus can be made confluent with the atrial septal defect, which is almost invariably at the oval fossa. It is important to remove enough of the party wall to ensure that the patch placed across the orifice of the coronary sinus and oval fossa does not produce obstruction at the

site of the incised sinus septum (Fig. 8.7).

The second problematic type of connexion is the infradiaphragmatic variant. The extrapericardial common pulmonary venous trunk is further from the posterior left atrial wall than might be expected. Because of this, the anastomosis effected between the trunk and left atrium is vulnerable to obstruction, particularly at its lateral extreme. This may become evident only when bypass is discontinued and the heart fills with blood.

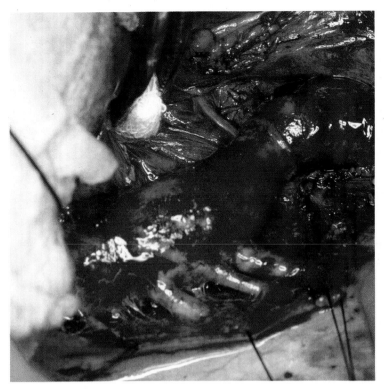

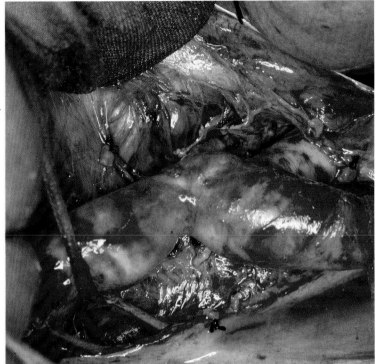

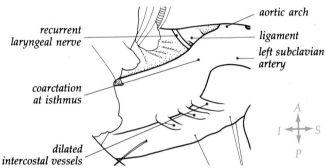

Fig. 8.8 *Operative view through a left thoracotomy of a coarctation with enlarged intercostal arteries, part of a well developed collateral circulation.*

Fig. 8.9 *Operative view through a left thoracotomy of a coarctation without a well developed collateral circulation.*

iii. Anomalies of the aorta

The congenital anomalies of the thoracic aorta which are of interest to the surgeon include coarctation, the spectrum of partial to complete interruption of the aorta, and vascular 'rings'. For this discussion, a coarctation is defined as a congenitally-derived discrete shelf-like lesion within the aorta which causes obstruction to blood flow. It is most often found just distal to the left subclavian artery but can occur proximally or more distally and even in the abdominal aorta. It is usually accompanied by some degree of tubular hypoplasia of the aorta but is anatomically independent of the hypoplasia. Its presence may be linked with other lesions associated with diminished left-sided flow, but coarctation can and does occur independently. We prefer to consider tubular hypoplasia one extreme of a spectrum leading to atresia or interruption of the aortic arch (*Becker & Anderson, 1981*).

Much has been made of the role of ductal tissue in the aetiology of coarctation. This subject has been recently reviewed (*Ho & Anderson, 1979*) and will

not be discussed further. The significant features of the duct devolve upon its patency. If the duct is patent, almost invariably there is an associated congenital anomaly which promotes increased blood flow through the pulmonary trunk and diverts blood away from the proximal aorta. In these circumstances the associated anomaly tends to dominate the picture and to determine the most appropriate surgical therapy. On the other hand, coarctation with a closed duct is very likely to be an isolated lesion, except for the occasional association with a bicuspid aortic valve (*Becker, Becker & Edwards, 1970*).

The chief concerns of the surgeon relate to the specific anatomy of the coarctation. The nature of the collateral circulation is of particular significance. With well developed collateral arteries (Fig. 8.8) there is little danger of cross-clamping the aorta during repair. However, if the collaterals are less well developed (Fig. 8.9), clamping the aorta may have several deleterious consequences. These include left ventricular strain due to proximal hypertension, which may also

induce a cerebrovascular accident secondary to rupture of a 'berry' aneurysm. There may be distal aortic hypotension (less than 50mm mercury pressure) which endangers the splanchnic and spinal vascular beds. Irrespective of the nature of the collaterals, the spinal circulation is best preserved by interrupting none or as few as possible of the intercostal vessels. Temporary occlusion of the intercostal vessels adjacent to the operative field seems to be a reasonable compromise in this difficult situation.

A final noteworthy feature is an anomalous artery, sometimes referred to as 'Abbott's artery', which may arise from the posteromedial aspect of the proximal descending aorta. Whether this is an enlarged bronchial artery or a 'persistence of the evanescent fifth arch', as suggested by Hamilton and Abbott (1928), is irrelevant. What is important is that the surgeon be aware that this anomalous vessel does exist and can lead to substantial bleeding during coarctation repair if not properly managed (*Lerberg, 1982*).

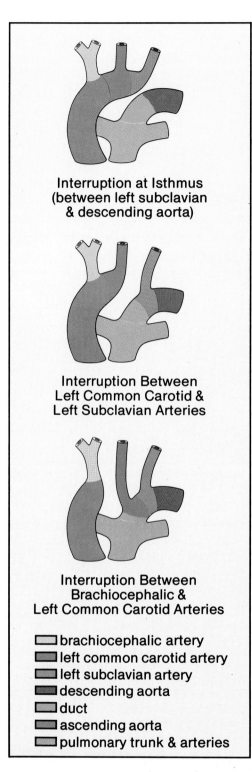

Interruption at Isthmus
(between left subclavian
& descending aorta)

Interruption Between
Left Common Carotid &
Left Subclavian Arteries

Interruption Between
Brachiocephalic &
Left Common Carotid Arteries

☐ brachiocephalic artery
☐ left common carotid artery
☐ left subclavian artery
☐ descending aorta
☐ duct
☐ ascending aorta
☐ pulmonary trunk & arteries

Fig. 8.10 *Basic types of interrupted aortic arch. Each type can exist with retroesophageal origin of the right subclavian artery.*

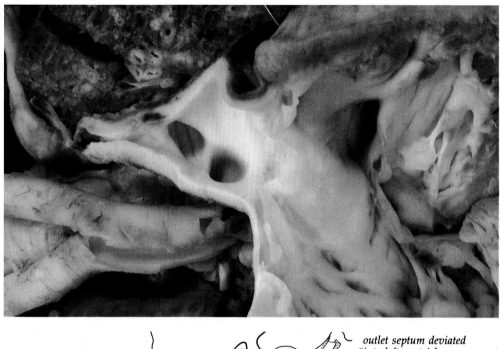

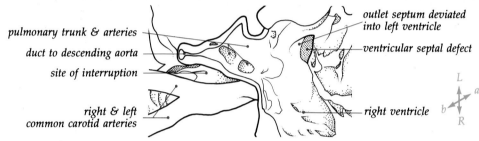

pulmonary trunk & arteries
duct to descending aorta
site of interruption
right & left common carotid arteries
outlet septum deviated into left ventricle
ventricular septal defect
right ventricle

Fig. 8.11 *Typical malalignment defect found in interruption of the aortic arch, in surgical orientation. The circulation to the lower body is duct-dependent.*

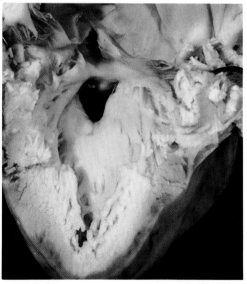

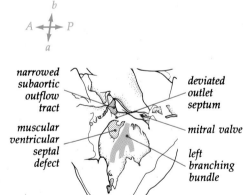

narrowed subaortic outflow tract
muscular ventricular septal defect
deviated outlet septum
mitral valve
left branching bundle

Fig. 8.12 *Anatomically orientated left ventricular aspect of a case of interrupted arch with deviated outlet septum narrowing the subaortic outflow tract.*

Discontinuity of the aorta, as opposed to coarctation, has been variously referred to as absence, atresia or interruption of the arch. Included in this group are those cases with a fibrous cord or bridge of tissue as well as those with a gap or absolute discontinuity at some point in the arch. Interruption can occur at one of three positions: at the isthmus; between the left subclavian and left common carotid arteries; and between the left common carotid and brachiocephalic arteries (Fig. 8.10). Almost invariably, these lesions are associated with a unilateral left aortic arch but, rarely, a

right arch can be similarly affected (*Pierpont et al., 1982*).

Since patients with discontinuity of the aorta are liable to early death (*Roberts, Morrow & Braunwald, 1962; Van Praagh et al., 1971*), they are a particular challenge to the clinician. The associated cardiovascular malformations are of critical importance since their very nature, perhaps more than the interrupted arch itself, affects the operative outcome. Almost always there is a patent connexion to the distal aorta through the duct (Fig. 8.11). A 'proximal' septal defect is also the rule. This is most frequently a

ventricular septal defect but occasionally an aortopulmonary window is found. The ventricular septal defect is usually perimembranous in association with posterior and leftward displacement of the infundibular septum, resulting in subaortic stenosis (Fig. 8.12). Any type of defect can be found, including on rare occasions those with anterior displacement which causes a Fallot-like obstruction to right ventricular outflow (*Ho et al., 1982*). Abnormal ventriculoarterial connexions are not unusual and present their own particular problems for operative reconstruction.

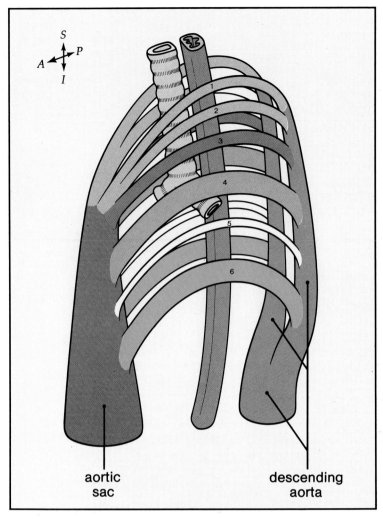

aortic
sac

descending
aorta

Fig. 8.13 *Pattern of bilateral aortic arch found during early development of the heart.*

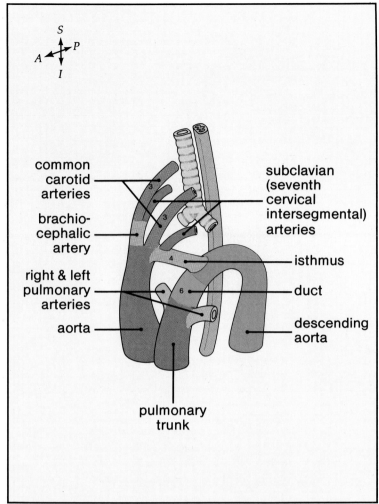

common
carotid
arteries

brachio-
cephalic
artery

right & left
pulmonary
arteries

aorta

pulmonary
trunk

subclavian
(seventh
cervical
intersegmental)
arteries

isthmus

duct

descending
aorta

Fig. 8.14 *The definitive left-sided aortic system derived from the originally bilaterally symmetrical arrangement.*

A less lethal but fairly frequently associated arterial abnormality is an aberrant right subclavian artery arising in retroesophageal position from the distal aorta. Since the arch is interrupted, symptoms of a vascular ring are unlikely unless a ring is created while reconstructing the arch. Conversely, if the aberrant artery is brought forward, it could be useful in repairing the aorta. This emphasizes the critical importance of clearly defining the nature and effect of associated abnormalities. Successful anatomical correction is as dependent on appropriate management of these accompanying lesions as it is on establishing aortic continuity.

Aortic rings are malformations associated with abnormal regression of part of a 'double aortic arch'. Knowledge of the development of the aortic arches is a genuine aid to understanding the morphology of these anomalies, although it is undesirable to use embryological hypothesis as proven fact. Of the six pairs of aortic arches connecting the anterior (ventral) and posterior (dorsal) aorta during development (Fig. 8.13), only the third, fourth and sixth arches remain recognizable in the postnatal heart. Most often, remnants of the third arch supply

the head; the fourth becomes part of the definitive aortic arch, and the left sixth arch becomes the duct (Fig. 8.14). The subclavian arteries, which are the seventh cervical intersegmental arteries, come to take origin from the fourth arch between the third and sixth arches when the heart migrates inferiorly (*Barry, 1951*). The hypothetical double aortic arch (*Stewart, Kincaid & Edwards, 1964*) consists of a midline anterior aorta which connects the bilateral fourth arches and bilateral posterior aortic segments to a midline descending aorta (Fig. 8.15). The fourth arches give rise to the remnants of the third arch and the bilateral sixth arches. Initially the arterial system is bilaterally symmetrical and the arches encircle the gut. Then, normally during early development, the entire right arch distal to the right third arch regresses, leaving a left arch and a left-sided aorta (Fig. 8.14). Failure of this regression leads to various forms of a 'ring' around the trachea and oesophagus. Most malformations of this nature are associated with a right aortic arch.

Not only can persistent patency of an aortic ring cause problems, but inappropriate interruption or atresia of part of the ring may result in abnormal

anatomy. Such a situation is illustrated in Fig. 8.16, which shows a left aortic arch with an aberrant right subclavian artery and bilateral ducts. In the scheme of Stewart et al. (1964), this anomaly would be placed in subgroup IIB3. Our preference is for descriptive analysis rather than alphanumeric notation. It should be noted that, as in the latter example of focal atresia, the atretic segment may not persist as a fibrous cord and may not necessarily cause compression of the trachea or oesophagus. Also, the size of the component parts of the ring is at least as important in producing symptoms as the particular anatomic arrangement. This accounts for the high incidence of symptoms associated with double aortic arch. Indeed, when only a fibrous cord is found, compression is not always apparent. Fig. 8.17 (left) shows a duct attaching the left pulmonary artery to an aberrant left subclavian artery which arises from a right arch (Fig. 8.17, centre). The considerable tracheoesophageal compression is not obvious until the duct is divided and its ends allowed to retract (Fig. 8.17, right). A detailed description of the various combinations of aortic rings can be found in the atlas by Stewart et al. (1964).

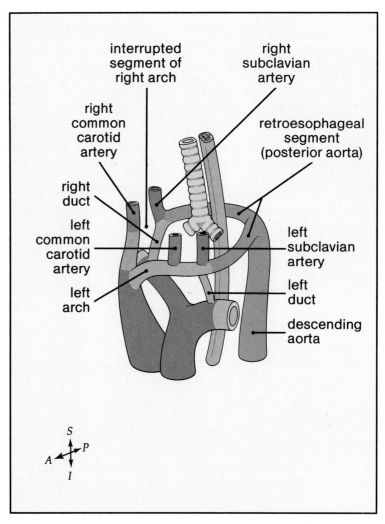

Fig. 8.15 *Hypothetical double aortic arch system based on the developmental pattern in Fig. 8.13 which provides the basis for understanding aortic rings.*

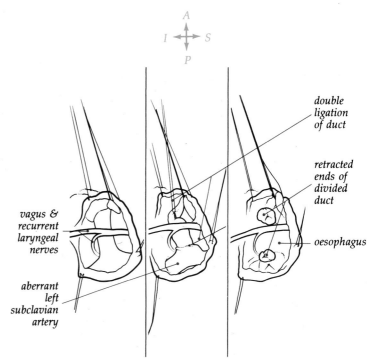

Fig. 8.16 *Left aortic arch with aberrant right subclavian artery and bilateral duct can be interpreted in terms of the hypothetical double arch.*

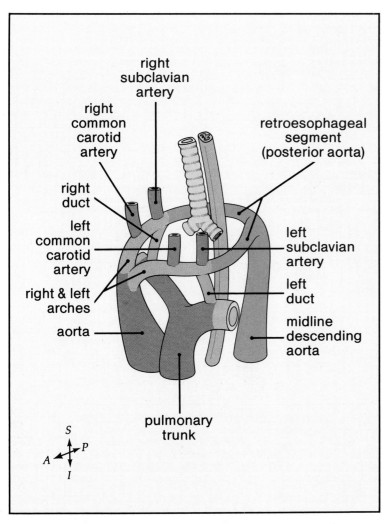

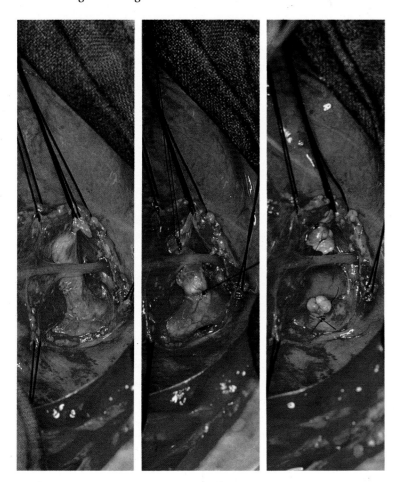

Fig. 8.17 *Operative views through a left thoracotomy of a duct connecting a right aortic arch to an aberrant left subclavian artery (left & centre); after division of the duct, the ends spring apart to free the oesophagus (right).*

8.9

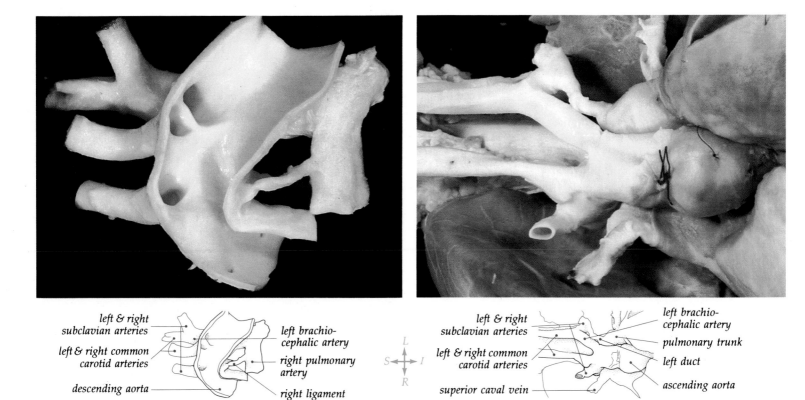

Fig. 8.18 *Surgically orientated (as for a median sternotomy) mirror-image branching pattern of the head and neck arteries in a right aortic arch.*

Fig. 8.19 *Right aortic arch with a left-sided duct, in surgical (median sternotomy) orientation.*

A word must be said about the right-sided aortic arch apart from its association with vascular ring abnormalities. A right-sided aortic arch is defined as one which crosses over the right main stem bronchus. It may connect to a descending aorta on either the right or left side of the vertebral column. A right-sided aortic arch is considered abnormal with the usual atrial arrangement, but in patients with the mirror-image arrangement it is 'normal'. In either it may or may not produce problems clinically. Its chief surgical significance lies in its association with about one-fourth of cases of tetralogy of Fallot and approximately half of all patients with common arterial trunks.

When subclavian-pulmonary artery shunts are contemplated, it is important to recognize that in patients with a right aortic arch one usually finds a mirror-image arrangement of the head, neck and arm arteries (Fig. 8.18). The first branch of the aorta beyond the coronaries is a brachiocephalic trunk which gives rise to the left subclavian and common carotid arteries. Under such circumstances the surgeon may elect a left-sided anastomosis to avoid kinking of the right subclavian artery as it is turned down into the mediastinum. However, the duct is usually a left-sided structure connecting the brachiocephalic trunk to the left pulmonary artery (Fig. 8.19). Perhaps because of this mirror-image arrangement it is unusual for the subclavian artery to have an aberrant origin and, thus, under these circumstances it is equally unusual to find a symptomatic vascular ring.

iv. Pulmonary artery anomalies

By far the most common malformation of the pulmonary arteries, excluding atresia or stenosis, is for either the right or left pulmonary artery to have an aortic origin. Most frequently the anomalous artery arises from a duct. Although seen in the presence of pulmonary atresia, usually with the other lung supplied by major aortopulmonary collateral arteries, it can be found with the other pulmonary artery connected to the patent pulmonary trunk. In this arrangement often the duct will close with time and there will be apparent unilateral absence of the pulmonary artery initially fed through the duct. This is common in tetralogy of Fallot or double outlet right ventricle, but about half of the cases have otherwise normal hearts (*Pool, Vogel & Blount, 1962*). In our experience it is rare to find true absence of the hilar pulmonary artery.

Less frequently the anomalous pulmonary artery, usually the right, can arise directly from the ascending aorta (Fig. 8.20). Sometimes termed a 'hemitruncus', we cannot advocate use of this term since almost always there are two normally formed arterial valves, one which is aortic and the other guarding the pulmonary trunk supplying the normally connected pulmonary artery. Rarely, with a common arterial trunk the right pulmonary artery may take an unusually high origin from the right side of the ascending portion of the trunk. Still we would rather not call this 'hemitruncus', preferring the descriptive title of 'common trunk with anomalous origin of the right

pulmonary artery'.

When the anomalously connected pulmonary artery arises directly from the aorta, surgical repair consists simply of detachment from the aorta and reattachment to the pulmonary trunk. This is somewhat more difficult in the presence of a common trunk but the same basic principle is followed for repair. However, when the anomalous pulmonary artery is fed through a duct or connected by a ligament, it will arise from the aortic arch or a brachiocephalic artery. Care must then be taken during surgical reconstruction to ensure that ductal tissue is not incorporated with the anastomosis, since it may subsequently constrict and stenose the site of repair. It should be remembered that, in cases with unilateral absence of a pulmonary artery, it is usual to find pulmonary hypertension and pulmonary hypertensive vascular disease in the normally connected lung, probably because of its being disproportionately small and having to receive the entire right ventricular output (*Pool et al., 1962*).

A much rarer anomaly of the pulmonary arteries is when the left pulmonary artery arises from the right pulmonary artery. The abnormal left pulmonary vessel courses from the right chest and passes between the trachea and oesophagus to the left pulmonary hilum, creating a so-called 'vascular sling' (*Contro et al., 1958*; Fig. 8.21). This may result in repeated respiratory problems requiring division and transplantation of the offending artery. As discussed above, the right pulmonary artery may arise

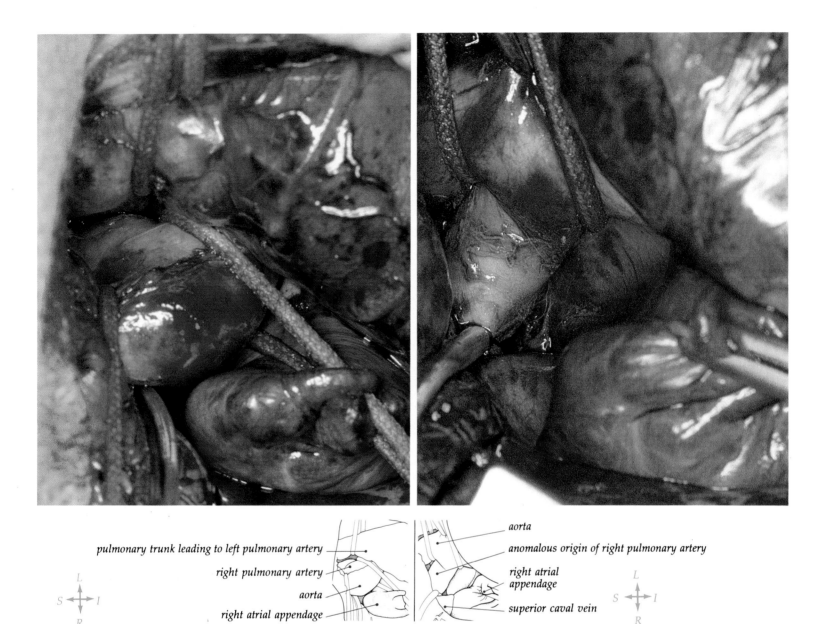

Fig. 8.20 *Operative views of an anomalous right pulmonary artery: (left) arising from the posterior aspect of the proximal aorta. Note its complete absence from the well developed pulmonary trunk;* *(right) coursing from its aortic origin to the right lung behind the superior caval vein.*

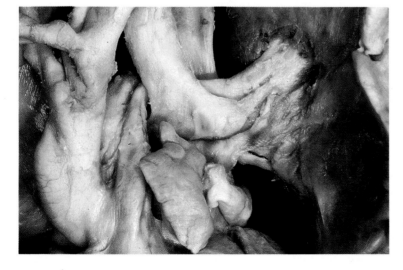

Fig. 8.21 *Origin of the left pulmonary artery from the right pulmonary artery with tracheal compression, a so-called vascular sling, in anatomical orientation. By courtesy of Prof. A. E. Becker.*

anomalously from the aorta or brachiocephalic artery; but an abnormal right pulmonary vessel arising from the left pulmonary artery has not, to our knowledge, been reported. The reason for this is not clear.

In the rare occurrence of agenesis of the right lung, displacement of the heart into the right chest may create a ring-like disposition which can obstruct the left bronchus. The displaced heart, pulling on the left pulmonary artery, draws the ligament and descending aorta across the left bronchus, compressing the bronchus against the spinal column. Division of the ligament and grafting of the aorta may be necessary to allow the pulmonary artery and aorta to spring apart and 'unroof' the constricting circle (*Maier & Gould, 1953; Harrison & Hendren, 1975; Harrison et al., 1980*).

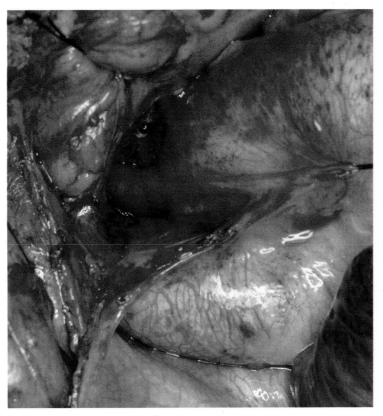

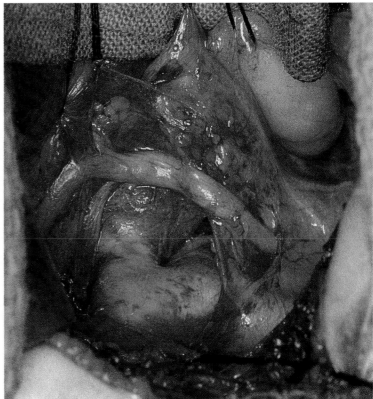

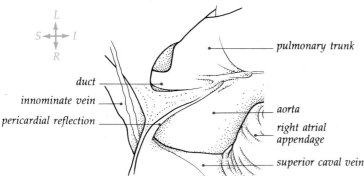

pulmonary trunk

duct
innominate vein
pericardial reflection

aorta
right atrial
appendage
superior caval vein

Fig. 8.22 *Operative view through a median sternotomy of a patent duct.*

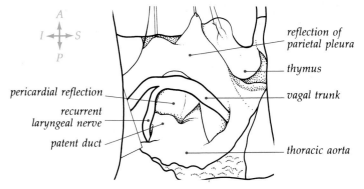

reflection of
parietal pleura

thymus

pericardial reflection
recurrent
laryngeal nerve
patent duct

vagal trunk

thoracic aorta

Fig. 8.23 *Operative view through a left lateral thoracotomy of a patent duct.*

v. Persistent duct and aortopulmonary window

Persistent duct occupies a special place in the study of cardiovascular disease since it was the first congenital heart lesion to be cured by operative intervention (*Gross, 1939*). Though it has recently been subject to various medical manoeuvres (*Starling & Elliott, 1974; Heymann, Rudolph & Silverman, 1976*), its interruption remains a paradigm of the best of surgical science. The anatomy is almost always predictable and the operative results uniformly excellent.

Since the arterial system develops with bilateral symmetry, a persistent duct may be either right- or left-sided, although the latter is overwhelmingly more common. Because the duct can persist on either side or bilaterally, it may be important in vascular ring anomalies. Also, persistent patency may play an important physiological role when it accompanies other complex congenital cardiovascular anomalies such as interrupted arch, aortic or pulmonary valve atresia or complete

transposition. This section is concerned with the usual primary congenital condition of isolated left-sided persistent patent duct.

Although an anterior approach to a patent duct is possible and sometimes necessary (Fig. 8.22), the normal operative approach is through a left lateral thoracotomy (Fig. 8.23). The duct arises from the posterosuperior aspect of the junction of the pulmonary trunk and left pulmonary artery. It courses posteriorly and slightly leftward to join the junction of the aortic arch and descending aorta just distal to and opposite the left subclavian orifice. Its pulmonary end is covered by a fold of pericardium and its aortic end by parietal pleura. Particularly in the infant it may be confused with the aortic isthmus; the left pulmonary artery may also be erroneously identified as a patent duct. Even under the best conditions, these other structures may be mistakenly ligated in lieu of the duct. The caveats of this procedure have recently been

elegantly reviewed by Pontius et al. (1981). Approached laterally, the best anatomical guide to the duct is the vagus nerve and its recurrent laryngeal branch. The vagus nerve passes along the subclavian artery and over the aortic arch before heading in a posterior direction to disappear behind the hilum. Just at the level of the duct it gives off the recurrent nerve (Fig. 8.24), which curves beneath the inferomedial wall of the duct before ascending along the posteromedial aspect of the aorta into the groove between the trachea and oesophagus.

Access to the duct may be achieved by incising the mediastinal parietal pleura, either between the phrenic and vagus nerves or more posteriorly over the aorta itself. With either approach the recurrent nerve must be visualized to guard against direct trauma or traction injury. The fold of pericardium extending over the pulmonary end of the duct may be lifted away by sharp dissection. The posteromedial wall of the duct is firmly attached by another more fibrous

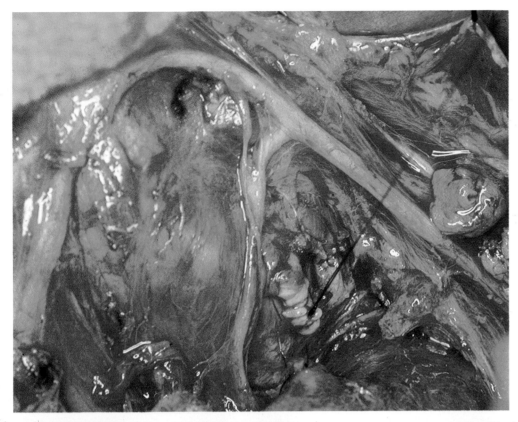

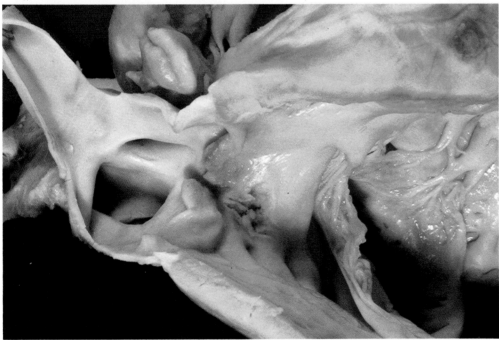

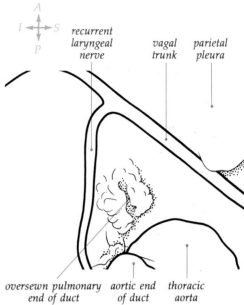

Fig. 8.24 *Operative view of the same heart as in Fig. 8.23 showing the relation of the recurrent laryngeal nerve to the site of the duct.*

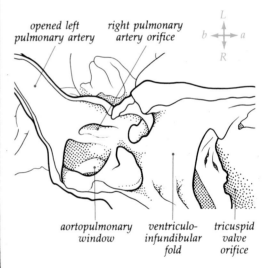

Fig. 8.25 *Large aortopulmonary window seen from its pulmonary trunk aspect, in surgical orientation.*

bronchus. It is this firm fibrous fold that prevents easy circumscription of the duct with a right-angle clamp. To minimize the risk of tearing the wall of the duct, this tissue must be divided by sharp dissection. This can be done through a superior approach over the aortic end of the duct or by freeing the aorta and retracting it medially. In the latter instance, small but potentially troublesome bronchial vessels may be encountered, arising from the posterior wall of the aorta. Another anatomical note of caution involves the thoracic duct and its tributaries in the area of the origin of the subclavian artery. Division of any of these major lymph vessels is liable to lead to chylothorax and its attendant

difficulties. Should the lymphatic trunks be inadvertently divided, they must be ligated to avoid chylothorax.

The duct in an infant or small child can measure 2–15mm in length and diameter. Rarely, one may encounter aneurysmal dilation of a duct (*Mendel, Luhmer & Oelert, 1980*). These may be aneurysms of a truly patent duct or may be simply a dilated ductal diverticulum with a closed pulmonary end. In general, the short 'fat' duct should be cross-clamped, divided and oversewn to minimize the chances of incomplete ligation or tearing of the vessel wall. For the longer 'thin' duct, a triple ligation technique has proved to be safe and effective (*Wilcox & Peters, 1967*).

The clinical presentation of aortopulmonary window is often similar to that of common trunks. The anatomical distinction lies in the ventriculoarterial connexion; where in a common trunk there is a single valve, aortopulmonary window is always associated with separate aortic and pulmonary valves. Though the ventricular septum is usually intact, this defect is frequently associated with additional congenital cardiovascular anomalies (*Faulkner et al., 1974*).

The defect itself is usually located in the right lateral wall of the pulmonary trunk anterior and opposite to the origin of the right pulmonary artery (Fig. 8.25). This means that its opening into the left side of

8.13

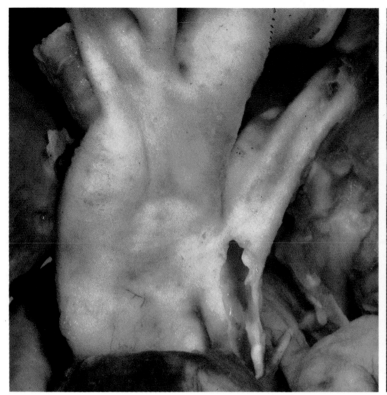
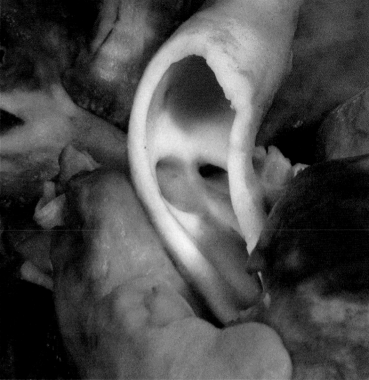

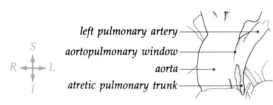

left pulmonary artery

aortopulmonary window

aorta

atretic pulmonary trunk

S
R ← → L
I

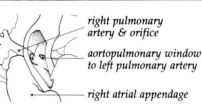

right pulmonary artery & orifice

aortopulmonary window to left pulmonary artery

right atrial appendage

S
R ← → L
I

Fig. 8.26 *Pulmonary atresia and ventricular septal defect with the right pulmonary artery arising directly from the aorta and the left pulmonary artery (left) connected to the atretic pulmonary trunk and (right) fed through an aortopulmonary window. By courtesy of Dr. J. L. Wilkinson & Mrs. A. Smith, University of Liverpool.*

the ascending aorta is just distal to the aortic bar and coronary arteries. The defect may appear as a well demarcated short tubular structure or it may be more like a window. Rarely, one pulmonary artery may arise directly from the aorta with a window leading to the pulmonary trunk and the other artery (Fig. 8.26). The surgical repair of aortopulmonary window is best accomplished through an incision in the ascending aorta using standard cardiopulmonary bypass techniques. As a general rule, 'closed' methods are not advisable, not even for the more tubular defects. Of course, when the window supplies a vital part of the circulation, it cannot be closed without providing an alternate source of blood for the dependent segment of the circulation.

Anderson, R.C., Heilig, W., Novick, R. & Jarvis, C. (1955) Anomalous inferior vena cava with azygous drainage: so-called absence of the inferior vena cava. *American Heart Journal*, **49**, 318–322.

Bankl, H. (1977) *Congenital Malformations of the Heart and Great Vessels*, p 194. Baltimore-Munich: Urban & Schwarzenberg.

Barry, A. (1951) Aortic arch derivatives in the human adult. *Anatomical Record*, **111**, 221–238.

Becker, A.E. & Anderson, R.H. (1981) *Pathology of Congenital Heart Disease*, pp 319–338. London: Butterworths.

Becker, A.E., Becker, M.J. & Edwards, J.E. (1970) Anomalies associated with coarctation of the aorta. Particular reference to infancy. *Circulation*, **41**, 1067–1075.

Bharati, S. & Lev, M. (1973) Congenital anomalies of the pulmonary veins. *Cardiovascular Clinics*, **5**, 23–41.

Contro, S., Miller, R.A., White, H. & Potts, W.J. (1958) Bronchial obstruction due to pulmonary artery anomalies. 1. Vascular sling. *Circulation*, **17**, 418–423.

DeLisle, G., Ando, M., Calder, A.L., Zuberbuhler, J.R., Rochenmacher, S., Alday, L.E., Mangino, O., Van Praagh, S. & Van Praagh, R. (1976) Total anomalous pulmonary venous connection: report of 93 autopsied cases with emphasis on diagnostic and surgical considerations. *American Heart Journal*, **91**, 99–122.

Edwards, J.E. & DuShane, J.W. (1950) Thoracic venous anomalies. I. Vascular connection between the left atrium and the left innominate vein (levoatriocardinal vein) associated with mitral atresia and premature closure of the foramen ovale (case 1). II. Pulmonary veins draining wholly to the ductus arteriosus (case 2). *Archives of Pathology*, **49**, 517–537.

Faulkner, S.L., Oldham, R.R., Atwood, G.F. & Graham, T.P. (1974) Aortopulmonary window, ventricular septal defect and membranous pulmonary atresia with a diagnosis of truncus arteriosus. *Chest*, **65**, 351–353.

Gross, R.E., (1939) Surgical management of patent ductus arteriosus with summary of four surgically treated cases. *Annals of Surgery*, **110**, 321–356.

Hamilton, W.F. & Abbott, M.E. (1928) Coarctation of the aorta of the adult type: Part I Complete obliteration of the descending arch at insertion of the ductus in a boy of fourteen; bicuspid aortic valve; impending rupture of the aorta; cerebral death. Part II A statistical study and historical retrospect of 200 recorded cases, with autopsy, of stenosis or obliteration of the descending arch in subjects above the age of two years. *American Heart Journal*, **3**, 381–421.

Harrison, M.R., Heldt, G.P., Brasch, R.C., de Lorimier, A.A. & Gregory, G.A. (1980) Resection of distal tracheal stenosis in a baby with agenesis of the lung. *Journal of Pediatric Surgery*, **15**, 938–943.

Harrison, M.R. & Hendren, W.H. (1975) Agenesis of the lung complicated by vascular compression and bronchomalacia. *Journal of Pediatric Surgery*, **10**, 813–817.

Heymann, M.A., Rudolph, A.M. & Silverman, N.H. (1976) Closure of the ductus arteriosus in premature infants by inhibition of prostaglandin synthesis. *New England Journal of Medicine*, **295**, 530–533.

Ho, S.Y. & Anderson, R.H. (1979) Coarctation, tubular hypoplasia and the ductus arteriosus: a histological study of 35 specimens. *British Heart Journal*, **41**, 268–274.

Ho, S.Y., Wilcox, B.R., Anderson, R.H. & Lincoln, C.R. (1982) Interrupted aortic arch. Anatomical features of surgical significance. *The Thoracic and Cardiovascular Surgeon*, **31**, 199–205.

Lerberg, D.B. (1982) Abbott's artery. *Annals of Thoracic Surgery*, **33**, 415–416.

Lucas, R.V.Jr., Woolfrey, B.F., Anderson, R.C., Lester, R.G. & Edwards, J.E. (1962) Atresia of the common pulmonary vein. *Pediatrics*, **29**, 729–739.

Maier, H.C. & Gould, W.J. (1953) Agenesis of the lung with vascular compression of the tracheobronchial tree. *Journal of Pediatrics*, **43**, 38–42.

Mendel, V., Luhmer, J. & Oelert, H. (1980) Aneurysma des Ductus arteriosus bei einem Neugeborenen. *Herz*, **5**, 320–323.

Moller, J.H., Nakib, A., Anderson, R.C. & Edwards, J.E. (1967) Congenital cardiac disease associated with polysplenia: A developmental complex of bilateral 'left-sidedness'. *Circulation*, **36**, 789–799.

Mortensson, W. & Lundstrom, N.R. (1974) Congenital obstruction of the pulmonary veins at their junctions. Review of the literature and a case report. *American Heart Journal*, **87**, 359–362.

Nakib, A., Moller, J.H., Kanjuh, V.I. & Edwards, J.E. (1967) Anomalies of the pulmonary veins. *American Journal of Cardiology*, **20**, 77–90.

Neill, C.A., Ferencz, C., Sabiston, D.C. & Sheldon, H. (1960) The familial occurrence of hypoplastic right lung with systemic arterial supply and venous drainage 'scimitar syndrome'. *The Johns Hopkins Medical Journal*, **107**, 1–15.

Pierpont, M.E.M., Zollikofer, C.L., Moller, J.H. & Edwards, J.E. (1982) Interruption of the aortic arch with right descending aorta. *Pediatric Cardiology*, **2**, 153–159.

Pontius, R.G., Danielson, G.K., Noonan, J.A. & Judson, J.P. (1981) Illusions leading to surgical closure of the distal left pulmonary artery instead of the ductus arteriosus. *Journal of Thoracic and Cardiovascular Surgery*, **82**, 107–113.

Pool, P.E., Vogel, J.H.K. & Blount, S.G.Jr. (1962) Congenital unilateral absence of a pulmonary artery. The importance of flow in pulmonary hypertension. *American Journal of Cardiology*, **10**, 706–732.

Roberts, W.C., Morrow, A.G. & Braunwald, E. (1962) Complete interruption of the aortic arch. *Circulation*, **26**, 39–59.

Starling, M.B. & Elliott, R.B. (1974) The effect of prostaglandins, prostaglandin inhibition, and oxygen on the closure of the ductus arteriosus, pulmonary arteries, and umbilical vessels in vitro. *Prostaglandins*, **8**, 187–203.

Stewart, J.R., Kincaid, O.W. & Edwards, J.E. (1964) *An Atlas of Vascular Rings and Related Malformations of the Aortic Arch System*. Springfield: Charles C Thomas.

Van Praagh, R., Bernhard, W.P., Rosenthal, A., Parisi, L.F. & Fyler, D.C. (1971) Interrupted aortic arch: surgical treatment. *American Journal of Cardiology*, **27**, 200–211.

Venables, A.W. (1963) Isolated drainage of the inferior vena cava to the left atrium. *British Heart Journal*, **25**, 545–548.

Wilcox, B.R. & Peters, R.M. (1967) The surgery of patent ductus arteriosus: a clinical report of 14 years' experience without an operative death. *Annals of Thoracic Surgery*, **3**, 126–131.

Winter, F.S. (1954) Persistent left superior vena cava: survey of world literature and report of 30 additional cases. *Angiology*, **5**, 90–132.

9 Positional Anomalies of the Heart

The surgical problems posed by cardiac malformations may be considerably increased when the heart itself is in an abnormal position. This is in part due to the unusual anatomical perspective presented to the surgeon because of the malposition, and also to the abnormal locations of the cardiac chambers which may necessitate approaches other than those already discussed. It is vital to stress that cardiac malposition is not in itself a diagnosis. Any normal or abnormal segmental combination can be found in an abnormally located heart. The heart itself may be normal, despite the malposition, but frequently, extremely complex anomalies are present. Consequently, the very presence of an abnormal cardiac position emphasizes the need for a full and detailed segmental analysis of the heart. All the rules enunciated in Chapter 5 certainly apply when the heart is not in its anticipated position. In this chapter, therefore, we confine ourselves to a description of malpositioned hearts and a detailed discussion of specific types of malposition. We conclude with a brief review of the surgical significance of atrial isomerism, which is generally held to be one of the major harbingers of abnormal cardiac position (*Van Praagh et al., 1964*).

When describing an abnormally located heart it is necessary to take account of its position within the chest and the direction of its apex. It is thus necessary to define normality. In the normal individual the heart is positioned with its apex to the left and two-thirds of its bulk to the left of the midline. A mirror-image atrial arrangement usually accompanies a mirror-image cardiac arrangement, that is, the apex points to the right with the greater part of the cardiac mass in the right hemithorax. With atrial isomerism, however, there is no norm. Thus, for all patients with atrial isomerism and those with the usual or mirror-image atrial arrangements and abnormally positioned hearts, it is necessary to have a system to describe cardiac malposition. In the past, formidable conventions have been constructed using terms such as dextrocardia, dextroposition, dextrorotation and pivotal dextrocardia (see *Wilkinson & Acerete, 1973* for review). In practice the only requirement is a system which accounts for two major features: the position of the cardiac mass relative to the chest silhouette; and the direction of the cardiac apex. This is because cardiac position and apex orientation, although usually congruent, are not invariably linked together. Some systems, such as that proposed by a group including one of the present authors (*Calcaterra et al., 1979*), have defined dextrocardia as the heart in the right chest with the apex to the right. But what happens in the rare occasion that the heart is in the right chest with its apex to the left? According to the convention recommended in Chapter 5, this is readily

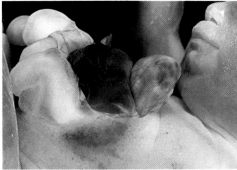

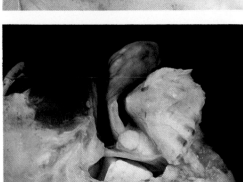

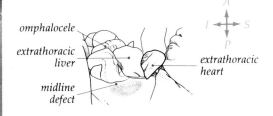

Fig. 9.1 *Thoracoabdominal ectopia cordis in a stillborn fetus. By courtesy of Dr. N. Fagg, Guy's Hospital, London.*

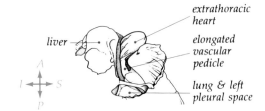

Fig. 9.2 *Further dissection of the fetus in Fig. 9.1 shows the elongated venous and arterial pedicles. By courtesy of Dr. N. Fagg, Guy's Hospital, London.*

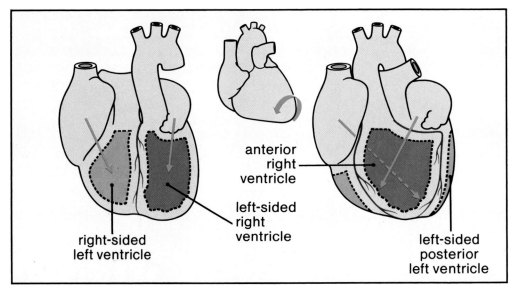

Fig. 9.3 *Rotation of a heart with atrioventricular discordance can change (left) the anticipated relationships of the ventricles to (right) a so-called 'criss-cross' relationship. The rotation is counter-clockwise, as from the apex.*

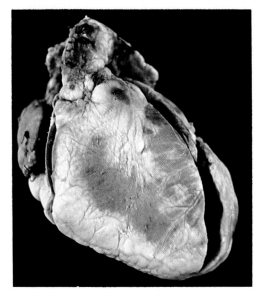

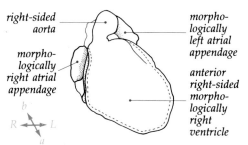

Fig. 9.4 *Anteroposterior view of a heart with an anterior right-sided aorta together with the usual atrial arrangement and the anticipated relationships for complete transposition.*

described as 'heart in right chest, apex to left', and we again endorse its value. Those who wish to give nominative definitions to the arrangement are free to do so, but we find the descriptive terms to be entirely adequate and less liable to misconstruction. Thus, the heart is described as being mostly in the left chest, right chest or midline, and the apical orientation is to the left, to the right or to the middle.

This description does not account for the most severe cardiac malposition, namely ectopia cordis. It has been said that the heart can be outside the thoracic cavity in cervical, thoracic, thoraco-abdominal or abdominal position. The review by Van Praagh and his colleagues (1983) questions the cervical and abdominal variants, classifying all cases as effectively thoracic or thoracoabdominal. In the thoracic type, which is the most common, there is a sternal defect and absence of the parietal pericardium. The heart protrudes directly from the thorax as illustrated in the classical case of Byron (1948). Usually there is an associated omphalocele and a small thoracic cavity. Such a case was successfully repaired in 1975 by Saxena, Koop and their colleagues in Philadelphia (see *Van Praagh et al., 1983*).

In the thoracoabdominal type, the sternal defect is usually confluent with abdominal wall and diaphragmatic defects, so the heart and various abdominal organs are displaced into an omphalocele (Fig. 9.1). Usually, this variant is associated with severe intracardiac malformations. For example, in the case shown in Fig. 9.1 there was tricuspid and pulmonary atresia. In this heart and in another with similar but less severe malformation that we examined recently, the venous components of both atria and the arterial trunks had been elongated because of the extrathoracic location of the heart (Fig. 9.2). These lengthy pedicles could well have produced problems with redundant tissue if operative correction had been attempted.

Our descriptive system also provides no information as to whether the unusual situation is a result of congenital malformation. For example, the heart may be in the right chest secondary to a pulmonary defect or because of gross enlargement of its right-sided chambers. In each case the problems of access presented to the surgeon are similar. Indeed, there is no reason for a patient with a lesion such as corrected transposition not to acquire a heart in the right chest because of pulmonary problems or right-sided hypertrophy.

There are certain lesions which readily spring to mind in connexion with hearts in the right chest and the usual atrial arrangement and with hearts in the left chest and mirror-image atria. The most notable of these is corrected

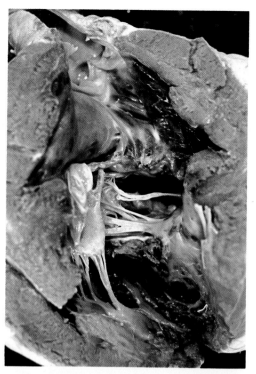

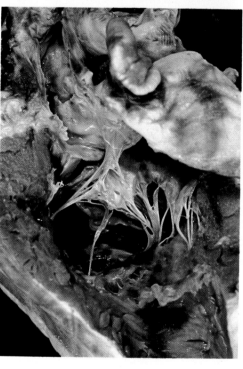

transposition (*Van Praagh et al., 1964*). An important point concerning patients with abnormally positioned hearts is that it is essential that the surgeon be aware of the locations of the chambers within the malpositioned organ so that the operation can be planned appropriately.

With the sophistication of modern diagnostic techniques it is unlikely that the surgeon will be presented with a patient with an abnormally located heart without a full preoperative diagnosis. There are, however, particular cardiac chamber arrangements which can still give major difficulties in diagnosis, notably the so-called 'criss-cross hearts' and 'superoinferior ventricles'. In these anomalies the ventricular relationships, or more rarely the ventricular topology (using the term 'topology' as defined in

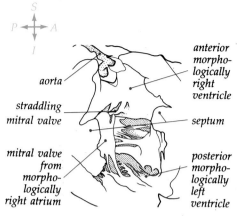

Fig. 9.5 *Opened right atrioventricular junction of the heart in Fig. 9.4. The right atrium is connected to a posterior morphologically left ventricle extending to the left. The right atrioventricular valve straddles and a catheter introduced through the right atrium could easily enter the anterior morphologically right ventricle.*

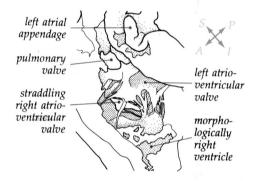

Fig. 9.6 *Further dissection shows that the morphologically right ventricle supports both the pulmonary trunk and aorta (see Fig. 9.5) though connected to the left atrium, and is anterior and right-sided because of rotation of the ventricular mass, in other words a 'criss-cross' heart. By courtesy of Drs. A.L. Moulton & M. Berman, University of Maryland, Baltimore.*

Chapter 5), are not as anticipated for a given atrioventricular connexion (*Anderson, 1982*). In a patient with corrected transposition and a 'criss-cross' arrange-ment, the morphologically right ventricle will be predominantly right-sided rather than in its anticipated left-sided position. This is a consequence of rotation of the ventricular mass in its long axis (Fig. 9.3). In addition to these unusual relationships, there is the possibility that a catheter passed through the right atrioventricular valve in a heart with atrioventricular discordance and 'criss-cross' relationships may slip through a ventricular septal defect and opacify the right-sided morphologically right ventricle. This will give the spurious appearance of atrio-ventricular concordance (*Symons et al., 1977*; Figs. 9.4 – 9.6).

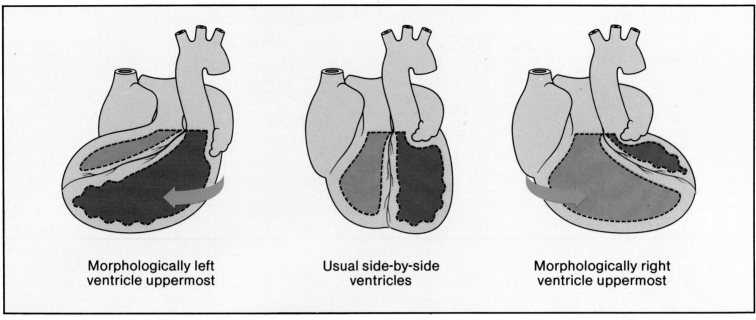

Morphologically left
ventricle uppermost

Usual side-by-side
ventricles

Morphologically right
ventricle uppermost

Fig. 9.7 *Tilting along the ventricular long axis produces so-called superoinferior ventricles, shown in the setting of atrioventricular discordance.*

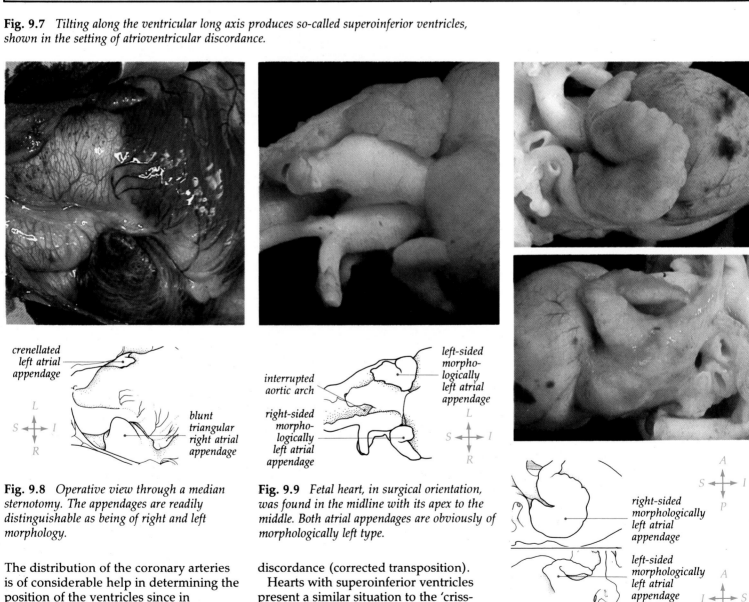

crenellated left atrial appendage

blunt triangular right atrial appendage

Fig. 9.8 *Operative view through a median sternotomy. The appendages are readily distinguishable as being of right and left morphology.*

interrupted aortic arch

right-sided morphologically left atrial appendage

left-sided morphologically left atrial appendage

Fig. 9.9 *Fetal heart, in surgical orientation, was found in the midline with its apex to the middle. Both atrial appendages are obviously of morphologically left type.*

right-sided morphologically left atrial appendage

left-sided morphologically left atrial appendage

Fig. 9.10 *Lateral views of the atrial appendages in Fig. 9.9 confirm that both are of morphologically left type. The diagnosis is left atrial isomerism. By courtesy of Dr. L. Allan, Guy's Hospital, London.*

The distribution of the coronary arteries is of considerable help in determining the position of the ventricles since in corrected transposition the anterior interventricular coronary artery arises from the right-sided coronary artery. Thus, in a heart which at first sight appears to be in complete transposition, finding the anterior interventricular artery with this disposition should alert the surgeon to the appropriate diagnosis of atrioventricular discordance (corrected transposition).

Hearts with superoinferior ventricles present a similar situation to the 'criss-cross' arrangement except that the heart is tilted along its long axis (Fig. 9.7). In some cases it is rotated as well as tilted so that both 'criss-cross' and superoinferior arrangements are present. Again the interventricular coronary arteries are useful because they indicate the plane of the ventricular septum and are excellent

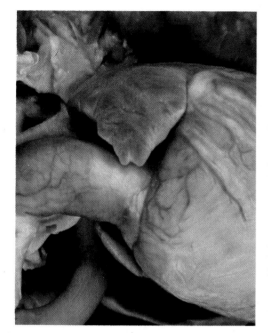
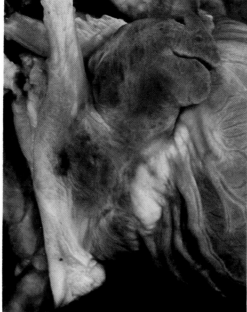
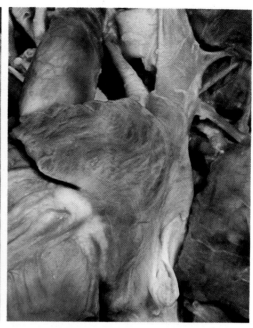

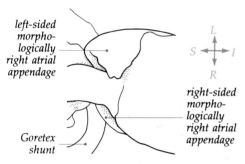

Fig. 9.11 *Heart in the right chest with its apex to the right, in surgical orientation. The left-sided atrial appendage is clearly of morphologically right type. The atrial arrangement must be either an inverted or a right isomeric type.*

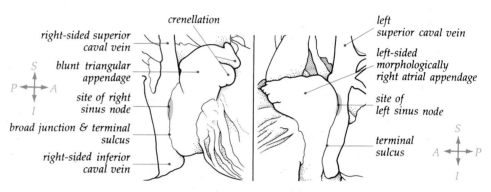

Fig. 9.12 *Lateral views of the atrial appendages in Fig. 9.11. Although the right-sided appendage is somewhat crenellated (left), its broad junction with the right-sided venous component and the large right superior caval vein indicates that it is of right morphology. The left-sided appendage is unequivocally of right morphology (right). Bronchial anatomy and bilateral terminal crests within the atria confirmed right atrial isomerism.*

guides to the position of the ventricular cavities. A point of consideration is that the distribution of the conduction tissue in these bizarre hearts is governed by the connexions of the chambers and not by the position of the chambers. These hearts are often further complicated by straddling and overriding atrioventricular valves. It is important to be aware that these abnormal relationships can be found with any combination of atrioventricular and ventriculoarterial connexions.

We have already mentioned the problems of atrial isomerism. Hearts with this atrial arrangement are not only found in unusual positions but are almost invariably associated with an abnormal arrangement of the thoracoabdominal viscera, hence the popular rubric of 'visceral heterotaxy'. It is still a widespread practice to classify these patients in terms of 'asplenia' and 'polysplenia' (*Stanger et al., 1977*). However, we believe that it is of greater value to base a system of categorization on atrial morphology. The first reason is that the splenic morphology

does not always correspond to the atrial anatomy. In our experience there is a greater correspondence between atrial anatomy and what is expected of the 'splenic syndrome' than between these syndromes and splenic morphology. Secondly and perhaps more importantly, it is of little consequence to the cardiac surgeon at operation whether his patient has one spleen, multiple spleens or no spleen at all. Use of atrial morphology to define these anomalies concentrates the attention upon the heart and enables the surgeon at operation to make immediately the diagnosis of atrial isomerism, even if this had not been predicted by the preoperative studies.

The atrial appendages are the best indicators of atrial morphology and can easily be distinguished as right or left type (Fig. 9.8). The surgeon must always confirm that his patient possesses lateralized atrial appendages. Left or right atrial isomerism (Figs. 9.9 – 9.12) is readily identifiable in autopsied hearts, and we believe that the finding of

isometric atrial appendages should put the surgeon on immediate alert.

In hearts with right atrial isomerism it is the rule to find complex intracardiac anomalies, usually with asplenia. There is total anomalous pulmonary venous connexion even if the pulmonary veins are connected to the heart. Almost always there are major anomalies of systemic venous drainage. A common atrioventricular valve is usually present, often with a univentricular atrioventricular connexion. Pulmonary stenosis or atresia is frequently found and the sinus nodes are bilateral (Fig. 9.12). Although operative experience with these hearts is increasing, the various combinations of anomalies militate against successful outcomes. To be forewarned is of great value, so it should be remembered that the best preoperative guide to isomerism is either cross-sectional ultrasonography of the abdominal great vessels (*Huhta, Smallhorn & Macartney, 1982*) or chest radiography of bronchial morphology (*Deanfield et al., 1980*).

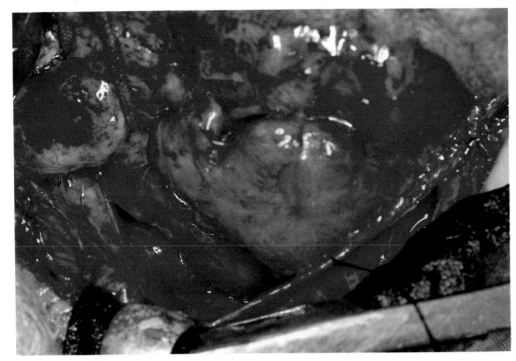

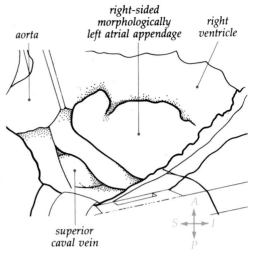

Fig. 9.13 *Operative view of a right-sided atrial appendage of morphologically left type. There was also azygos return of the inferior caval vein and double outlet right ventricle. The patient has left atrial isomerism.*

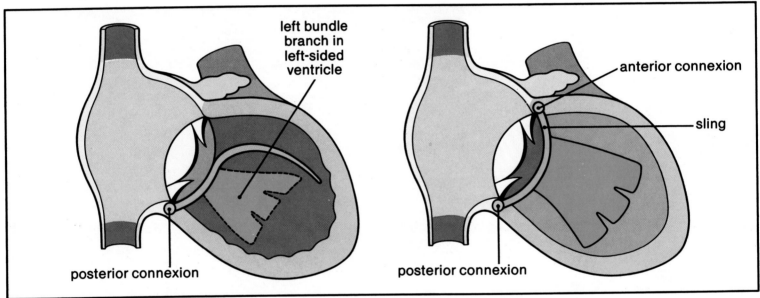

Fig. 9.14 *Anticipated conduction tissue disposition in biventricular atrioventricular connexion and atrial isomerism: (left) normal arrangement with a right-hand pattern of ventricular topology; (right) a sling with left-hand pattern of ventricular topology.*

Although right atrial isomerism is usually accompanied by severe intracardiac malformations, it is not always so with left atrial isomerism. Thus, the surgeon is more likely to be confronted with an undiagnosed case. It then becomes important to know that the sinus node is in an anomalous position. It is usually hypoplastic and, if it can be found, will be located close to the atrioventricular junction (*Dickinson et al., 1979*). Azygos return of the inferior caval vein is a frequent accompaniment (Fig. 9.13). In the more severely affected cases there may be a common atrioventricular valve. Pulmonary stenosis or atresia is not usually a feature, nor is the presence of a univentricular atrioventricular connexion.

Whatever the type of atrial isomerism, in the presence of a common valve with each atrium connected to its own ventricle, a left-hand pattern of ventricular topology

is frequently found. In this setting the heart may well be diagnosed as corrected transposition. However, the presence of atrial isomerism makes it highly likely that there will be a sling of conduction tissue. This places the entire edge of the ventricular septum at risk should surgical correction be attempted. When atrial isomerism is found with a biventricular

atrioventricular connexion and a right-hand pattern of ventricular topology, an atrioventricular conduction axis in its usual posterior position is to be anticipated (Fig. 9.14). Clearly this entire discussion emphasizes the significance of full sequential segmental analysis of any patient presented for cardiac surgery.

Anderson, R.H. (1982) Criss-cross hearts revisited. *Pediatric Cardiology*, **3**, 305–313.
Byron, F. (1948) Ectopia cordis. Report of a case with attempted operative correction. *Journal of Thoracic Surgery*, **17**, 717–722.
Calcaterra, G., Anderson, R.H., Lau, K.C. & Shinebourne, E.A. (1979) Dextrocardia – value of segmental analysis in its categorization. *British Heart Journal*, **42**, 497–507.
Deanfield, J., Leanage, R., Stroobant, J., Chrispin, A.R., Taylor, J.F.N. & Macartney, F.J. (1980) Use of high kilovoltage filtered beam radiographs for detection of bronchial situs in infants and young children. *British Heart Journal*, **44**, 577–583.
Dickinson, D.F., Wilkinson, J.L., Anderson, K.R., Smith, A., Ho, S.Y. & Anderson, R.H. (1979) The cardiac conduction system in situs ambiguus. *Circulation*, **59**, 879–885.
Huhta, J.C., Smallhorn, J.F. & Macartney, F.J. (1982) Two-dimensional echocardiographic diagnosis of situs. *British Heart Journal*, **48**, 97–108.
Symons, J.C., Shinebourne, E.A., Joseph, M.C., Lincoln, C.,

Ho, S.Y. & Anderson, R.H. (1977) Criss-cross heart with congenitally corrected transposition: report of a case with d-transposed aorta and ventricular preexcitation. *European Journal of Cardiology*, **5**, 493–505.
Stanger, P., Rudolph, A.M. & Edwards, J.E. (1977) Cardiac malpositions: an overview based on study of sixty-five necropsy specimens. *Circulation*, **56**, 159–172.
Van Praagh, R., Van Praagh, S., Vlad, P. & Keith, J.D. (1964) Anatomic types of congenital dextrocardia. Diagnostic and embryologic implications. *American Journal of Cardiology*, **13**, 510–531.
Van Praagh, R., Weinberg, P.M., Matsuoka, R. & Van Praagh, S. (1983) Malpositions of the Heart. In *Moss's Heart Disease in Infants, Children & Adolescents*, 3rd edition, pp 422–458. Edited by F.H. Adams & G.C. Emmanouilidas. Baltimore: Williams & Wilkins.
Wilkinson, J.L. & Acerete, F. (1973) Terminological pitfalls in congenital heart disease. Reappraisal of some confusing terms, with an account of a simplified system of basic nomenclature. *British Heart Journal*, **35**, 1166–1177.

Index